RELATIONSHIPS, SEX AND HEALTH EDUCATION 101

of related interest

What Does Consent Really Mean?
Pete Wallis and Thalia Wallis
Illustrated by Joseph Wilkins
ISBN 978 1 84819 330 7
eISBN 978 0 85701 285 2

Educating Young People About Pornography
Relationships and Sex Education (RSE) Activities for 11–19-year-olds
Vanessa Rogers
ISBN 978 1 78775 833 9
eISBN 978 1 78775 834 6

Going Beyond 'The Talk'
Relationships and Sexuality Education for those Supporting 12–18-year-olds
Sanderijn van der Doef, Clare Bennett and Arris Lueks
ISBN 978 1 78775 512 3
eISBN 978 1 78775 513 0

Talking Consent
16 Workshops on Relationship and Sex Education for Schools and Other Youth Settings
Thalia Wallis and Pete Wallis
ISBN 978 1 78775 081 4
eISBN 978 1 78775 082 1

Let's Talk Relationships
Activities for Exploring Love, Sex, Friendship and Family with Young People
Vanessa Rogers
ISBN 978 1 84905 136 1
eISBN 978 0 85700 340 9

RELATIONSHIPS, SEX AND HEALTH EDUCATION 101

Activity Toolkit for Working with Young People Aged 11+

KERRY CABBIN
Foreword by Dr Naomi Sutton

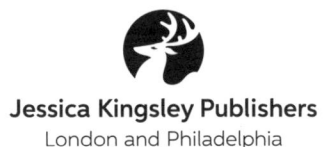

Jessica Kingsley Publishers
London and Philadelphia

First published in Great Britain in 2022 by Jessica Kingsley Publishers
An imprint of Hodder & Stoughton Ltd
An Hachette Company

1

 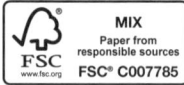
A CIP catalogue record for this title is available from the British Library and the Library of Congress

ISBN 978 1 78775 853 7
eISBN 978 1 78775 854 4

Printed and bound in Great Britain by Bell & Bain Limited

Jessica Kingsley Publishers' policy is to use papers that are natural, renewable and recyclable
products and made from wood grown in sustainable forests. The logging and manufacturing
processes are expected to conform to the environmental regulations of the country of origin.

Jessica Kingsley Publishers
Carmelite House
50 Victoria Embankment
London EC4Y 0DZ

www.jkp.com

MIX
Paper from
responsible sources
FSC
www.fsc.org   FSC® C007785

Contents

Foreword

I am a consultant physician and have been working in the area of sexual health for the last 14 years. In my day job, I work at Integrated Sexual Health Services at Rotherham Hospital but I am also known for my work as the TV Doctor on E4's series *The Sex Clinic*. Over the years working in sexual health, I have developed a professional and personal interest in the need for good quality relationships, sex and health education because too often I witness the correlation between a lack of education and poor sexual health outcomes. I regularly advocate in the media about the need to raise awareness of all things sexual health to reduce myths and misunderstandings and to promote communication about this topic.

I first came across Kerry through her amazing business Tough Cookies Education where she provides relationships and sex education (RSE) training, delivers workshops in schools across the country, and creates resources for educators and parents. I was instantly impressed by her passion for sex education. From our initial meeting via Twitter, I went on to support Kerry in promoting the work of Tough Cookies and we also delivered HIV awareness sessions together for teachers and youth workers.

Kerry's book is an approachable, flexible and easy-to-use resource which is a fantastic tool for anyone whose role it is to deliver relationships and sex education, whether this be in a classroom setting or out in the community. The book emphasizes the idea that sex education is more than just biology, and incorporates learning about peer pressure, effective communication, self-esteem, confidence building, and consent, alongside the topics of contraception and sexually transmitted infections. It provides information and inclusive teaching ideas, worksheets and activities which support you to be able to deliver good quality and effective RSE for young people aged 11+.

This carefully researched book has been written in an accessible manner and could be enjoyed as a single read-through or dipped into for information and strategies. Interwoven with examples from Kerry's own personal and professional experiences as a sex and relationships educator, this book is full of insights and practical tips which will be of great benefit to all who work to deliver relationships and sex education with children and young people.

Dr Naomi Sutton
Consultant Physician in Sexual Health and HIV

Acknowledgments

The chapters and activities in this book have been inspired and supported by the many young people and educators who have taken part in my relationships and sex education workshops, staff training, focus groups and Zooms! Thank you to my family, Dan, Laurie Elle and Remi for your continuous support and a special mention to Rekha Patel-Harrison for always being my sounding board for ideas.

Thank you to the local communities, schools and youth groups that have provided me with the space to practise and tweak the materials featured and for always sharing open and honest feedback with me, including Stephen Jackson, Droylsden Academy, Hayley Taylor, St Damian's RC Science College, Katherine France, The Queen Katherine and Ian Giles, Wardle Academy.

And thank you to all of the girls who took part in my Sunday sessions as part of the girls' group. Your evaluations and ideas have been invaluable.

Part 1

PREPARING TO TEACH RSE

• Chapter 1 •

Relationships, Sex and Education

First introduced in 2000, sex and relationships education or SRE as it was known (though the term later became RSE), was developed alongside the Labour government's teenage pregnancy strategy for England. The ten-year, national plan was established to halve the number of teenage conceptions and was supported by the implementation of a new and inclusive sex education programme. When I first began delivering SRE in schools, back then, the subject predominantly focused on delaying first-time sexual intercourse as well as encouraging condom use and working to support more young women to access young people's sexual health services and consider using long-acting reversible contraception. The programme was engrossed in teenage pregnancy, and I am pleased to see just how much the subject of SRE and the curriculum being delivered has now evolved over time.

Teaching about relationships and sex education (RSE) and health education now incorporates a wider variety of important youth-related topics such as puberty and period education, online relationships and digital safety, female genital mutilation (FGM), fertility, sexual harassment, sexuality, gender, healthy relationships and consent, to name just a few.

Many schools have been delivering aspects of RSE for some time, often as part of personal, social, health and economic education (PSHE) or via their character education and life skills programme, but for some schools the introduction of RSE provides an opportunity for them to create, design and deliver a brand-new subject.

Over the past five years, I have been working with a number of schools to help them devise their RSE curriculum plans. I have noticed a range of approaches to the introduction of RSE across education, from schools that have timetabled the subject, perhaps allocating a one-hour lesson per week, to others that have included it as part of life skills, or allocated space during form or tutorial times with drop-down days and year group assemblies scheduled to support this.

In September 2020, relationships, sex and health education became a mandatory subject for all schools in England to teach. Alongside the announcement of these changes, the Government shared new and updated statutory guidance for governing bodies, headteachers, principals, senior leadership teams and teachers. This was to replace the previous guidance on sex and relationships education from the Department for Education and Employment (2000).

The government guidance document provides teachers and others who have a responsibility for RSE with much needed, up-to-date advice and direction. Educators planning and delivering RSE and health education programmes will very quickly become familiar with this information, as it aims to steer and inform their relationships, sex and health education delivery plans and learning outcomes.

I often liken the RSE guidance to the recipe given during the technical challenge of *The Great British Bake Off* – a task where the instructions are limited or minimal, which encourages participants to use their own intuition and experience. For some subject leads, particularly those with vast experience of delivering RSE, this flexible guidance can be a positive introduction, as they can use their own initiative, ideas, training and experience, but for many, and particularly those educators new to teaching this fun and engaging topic, it can feel intimidating and stressful. This book aims to eliminate those feelings and provide educators with a go-to resource that can answer any questions and become an effective toolkit for the classroom.

The learning opportunities in this book aim to support the development of young people as they navigate their way through their teens and attempt to manage many first-time experiences. It will provide teaching ideas, activities and prompts, covering a range of RSE topics, developing young people's understanding, practising skills and exploring attitudes and opinions.

Effective programmes of relationships and sex education should include more than facts and figures. Good quality relationships and sex education should aim to support young people to build positive self-esteem and raise their confidence. It needs to provide reflective learning opportunities which can further develop their life skills and guide informed decision-making and healthy behaviour.

When delivered well, relationships, sex and health education can help to develop a young person's communication skills and provide great opportunities for them to reflect on their feelings about friendship and relationships. It develops young people's knowledge around health, wellbeing and their rights and responsibilities, and supports them to keep themselves and others safe.

> We want all children to grow up healthy, happy, safe, and able to manage the challenges and opportunities of modern Britain. That is why, from September 2020, all secondary age children will be taught Relationships, Sex and Health Education. (Department for Education 2020)

The group sessions and conversation opportunities facilitated as part of RSE lessons provide an open and honest safe space for young people to ask and obtain answers to many of their 'Am I normal?' questions about growing up, developing bodies, feelings and emotions, online safety, relationships and sex. The wider programme provides a pathway of learning which supports their resilience skills, confidence and feelings of empowerment as they journey through adolescence into adulthood.

Good RSE is a learning experience which a young person will remember. An important aspect of delivery will also require you to consider what you say in these lessons you teach and how you say it. It has been proven that this can also impact how young people will grow, think and feel about these life skills topics.

While working to provide workshops in schools, I have met many educators, including community and youth workers, youth offending team staff, pupil referral unit mentors and school-based staff such as RSE subject leads, form tutors and classroom assistants who are all working to improve relationships and sex education for young people having taken on their new role, developing programmes and teaching lessons which meet the requirements of the new government legislation. It is an exciting time for those with a keen interest in the subject.

As part of the new statutory offer, schools in England must also have in place a written policy for relationships and sex education. No policy is required for health education, which incorporates the learning outcomes for puberty and period education.

Government guidance states that schools in England should consult with parents and carers when developing and reviewing their relationships and sex education policy. It is also advised that the policy and plans respond to the needs of students and parents while reflecting the needs of the local community. The school's policy for relationships and sex education is required to be displayed on the school's website and should be made available to parents or carers on request.

Schools should consider ways in which they can effectively engage students in the planning and implementation of their RSE programmes too.

Giving students a voice encourages them to participate in, and eventually to own and drive, their learning. This means a complete shift from the traditional approach of teaching compliance that develops a 'learned helplessness' to an encouraging voice where there is authenticity in the learning.

Involving the voice of young people in the development and evaluation of RSE lets young people know that their expertise, opinions and ideas are valued. There are many ways in which a school can achieve this. For example:

- Setting up a student-led RSE steering group, providing a place where students can express their opinions and inform curriculum planning.
- Involving the student council in the development and creation of the RSE policy.
- Developing surveys and questionnaires to gather student feedback about the curriculum or about particular lessons and resources being used.
- Facilitating classroom discussions involving students in decision-making about age-appropriateness and when topics should be introduced and revisited.
- Working together with students to create classroom resources, fun learning materials, games, activities and posters.

Engaging with parents is another main focus of the new guidance, and there is reference made to this throughout the document. There is recognition of the important role parents play in educating their children, with the guidance stating that: 'Parents are the first teachers of their children. They have the most significant influence in enabling their children to grow and mature and to form healthy relationships' (Department for Education 2019).

Parents can be engaged a number of ways, both informally through day-to-day contact in the mornings and afternoons at drop-off and pick-up times, at the school gate and out and about in the community. They can be reached at after-school activities and through specific school events such as sports days, concerts, assemblies, fundraisers and social events, and more formally through stalls at open days, consultation events, and by providing adult learning opportunities. Like students, parents can take part in surveys, meetings and steering groups to inform and evaluate aspects of RSE.

As part of statutory RSE, parents have retained their right to request that their child be withdrawn from some or all of the sex education lessons being delivered. The guidance says that a parent's right to withdraw their child should be respected and encourages that a conversation takes place between a school representative and the parent to discuss and record this. The guidance also clarifies that in the final term before a young person turns 16, and if a young person wishes to receive sex education rather than be withdrawn, the school should make arrangements to provide this pupil with the sex education they have missed.

It is important for schools and educators to ensure that young people are made aware of their right to access these learning opportunities, and when planning your programme and delivery it would be a good idea to consider how you will inform young people of this, and how you will provide these learning opportunities should they be requested.

It has taken many years of campaigning from cross party-political groups, education unions, public health teams and third-sector organizations to get to a place where RSE and health education has become a mandatory subject. A wealth of evidence has been provided by many professionals working with young people to suggest why it is necessary.

The conclusion is that young people need better relationships, health and sex education and they need it now. It has to be accessible to all young people, including young people with special educational needs, and it is imperative that the programme is up to date and relevant to today's society. Curriculums, lesson plans and resources need to be revamped and ensure that the important, new and emerging topics such as grooming, FGM and gender are included.

It is also important that RSE is delivered at the right time, not too little and not too late. With the development of a primary relationships and health curriculum, young people should be able to follow a framework of learning that leads on from what they learned in their primary school setting.

In an ideal world, RSE should be provided by trained and informed staff who are passionate about the subject and want to inform and empower young people's health and relationships. Across the country an over-abundance of courses, including accredited, non-accredited, online and face to face, have become available. Currently in the UK, there are not any specific training standards for RSE. You will find lots of organizations and individuals offering guidance, support, development, learning materials and resources for delivering RSE. There are many learning opportunities offered both locally and nationally which would be beneficial to explore. And there is a wealth of topic-specific information available in this book.

◆ Chapter 2 ◆

Your Role as a Sex Educator

Over the past 20 years, communities, schools and classrooms have become much more diverse and I am happy to see that the new RSE curriculum has changed to include and respond to the varied needs of young people, diverse families and the wider community.

But the subject of relationships and sex education and the introduction of the many new topics can at times feel overwhelming, particularly for those of you who are new to teaching or new to the role of sex educator. So, before you begin planning and teaching relationships and sex education, it would be beneficial for you to recognize your own starting point and how you think and feel about the topics you will explore with young people.

This resource aims to inspire, empower, support and encourage you to provide a quality and effective programme of relationships, sex and health education. Part of achieving this is about considering and understanding your own development needs and recognizing why RSE and your role as a relationships and sex educator is crucial to supporting young people.

Delivering relationships, health and sex education can bring about personal challenges for facilitators, and many educators have expressed the concerns about their own lack of knowledge around the human body, genitalia, gender, sexuality, contraceptive choices and fertility. You are not required to be an expert on all of the topics, but a good understanding of the key facts and any laws and relevant news relating to the topics you are teaching would be helpful. Even more so, having the confidence to openly and honestly discuss and explore will be paramount to your role.

At the beginning of each subject area found in Part 2 of the book, you will find further information and guidance which will help you develop your understanding, knowledge and skills.

To eliminate any worries you may have about your role as sex educator, and to enable you to deliver an effective, relevant and enjoyable programme of RSE, it could be beneficial to set up and establish a local RSE network group. I have been involved in many such groups over the past 25 years and I have always found them to be beneficial for me and the young people and organization to which I provide services.

You may be the only lead for RSE in your school or organization, but by building a working group and RSE support network, which could include other members of staff from your school or organization, a school nurse, sexual health services, staff members from your local youth work team, faith leaders and parent representatives, you will be able to create opportunities where you can safely share your curriculum and teaching ideas and allow other members of staff and the community to evaluate, challenge and also offer support, which can be particularly useful if you are facing or likely to face any community or parental opposition.

Over the last few years, as schools began to prepare for statutory RSE, I encountered many good practice examples of this, where schools had brought together pastoral staff, safeguarding leads and heads of year, alongside parent representatives and community organizations, including young people's sexual health services, school nurses, and faith groups. These networks came together to plan, present and evaluate RSE work, as well as to share specialist skills and knowledge, and this led to successful and well-supported programmes of RSE and health education being designed and delivered.

Whether you are an RSE lead with the task of creating and developing a whole-school curriculum, providing schemes or work and teaching materials for others, or an educator with a focus on planning and designing assemblies and lessons for your own class, a good starting point before stepping into the classroom is to take some time to reflect on your own personal values with regards to relationships, sex and health education topics.

Our own personal values and life experiences, without us even being aware of it, will and can influence our session ideas, thoughts and delivery. They will inform the choices we make about what is relevant and age-appropriate and will guide the way we teach and talk about topics.

By taking the time to carry out these reflection activities you will be able to consider your own knowledge, skills, attitudes and opinions in relation to relationships and sex education and identify your personal strengths, weaknesses, areas for development and any further training needs.

RSE is a subject in which the activities themselves will include the exploration of values, attitudes and opinions, and so being aware of your own value base will be an important factor in planning and preparing to teach the subject and topics. When we reflect on and understand how our own experience and learning have impacted how we think and feel, we can ensure that the programmes we develop for RSE are free from our own unconscious biases and are inclusive to the young people and communities we serve.

Try out these quick and easy reflection activities to help prepare you to teach RSE.

YOUR SEX EDUCATION

- Think about your own sex education experience – whether this was delivered at school by a teacher, involved a talk at home from a parent, or maybe something you read in a book.
- Think carefully about the key messages you received from the sex education you experienced.
- Think openly about how the relationships, sex and health education you received made you feel, and what it made you think about relationships and love?

- Consider what your learning experiences taught you about your own changing body, growing up, sexuality and sex.

When we unpick the learning we have experienced about relationships, health and sex, we can better identify any messages which may be harmful or biased. This exercise also can help to identify where we have gaps in our knowledge and provide us with a plan of action to access and explore new learning opportunities.

To end this reflection activity, think about what you would like your students to say if they were asked this same question in years to come.

Understanding what you would like the final outcome to be can help you focus and find your starting point for planning.

This next activity can help you to identify which of the relationships, health and sex education topics lie outside your comfort zone. This can be carried out as an individual activity or with a team of educators.

LIKERT SCALE ACTIVITY

Draw a scale like the one below and using the list of relationships, sex and health education topics, place each topic on the scale to show how comfortable and/or how confident you feel with regards to talking about this topic with young people and about planning and delivering lessons about this.

If you have the space and are working with a team of educators, you can deliver the activity more interactively, reading out the topics and having the participants position themselves in the room, marking out clear spaces for comfortable and uncomfortable, confident and not at all confident and somewhere in between.

It is important when taking part in these activities to be completely open and honest about your inner thoughts and feelings and to not see any discomfort you may have about a particular topic or aspect of RSE as a weakness. This activity allows you to take action and make development plans which will enhance and improve your delivery and the experiences young people receive.

Likert scales you could use:

Not confident	Somewhat confident	Unsure	Confident	Very confident

Very uncomfortable	Uncomfortable	Neutral	Comfortable	Very comfortable

I have no knowledge of this topic	I have a little knowledge but need to learn more	I have some knowledge of this topic	I have good knowledge and could teach about it	I have excellent knowledge and could train others and create resources

List of relationships, sex and health education topics:

- Different types of relationships
- Same sex relationships
- Marriage and civil partnerships
- Respectful relationships
- Healthy intimate relationships
- Unhealthy relationships
- Ending relationships respectfully
- Gender stereotypes
- Bullying
- Cyberbullying
- Homophobic, biphobic and transphobic bullying
- The Equalities Act
- Sexuality
- Gender
- Sexual harassment
- Sexual violence
- Trusted adults
- Parenting
- Rights and responsibilities of digital citizens
- Risks of sharing online
- How to report online harmful material
- The impact of viewing harmful material online
- Sexually explicit material and pornography
- Criminal offences relating to the viewing and sharing of harmful material involving children, sexual consent
- Sexual exploitation
- Grooming
- Coercion
- Harassment
- Rape
- Domestic abuse
- Forced marriage
- Honour-based violence
- Female genital mutilation
- Sexual pressure
- Reproductive health, including fertility
- Delaying sex
- Contraceptive choices
- Pregnancy, including miscarriage
- Choices in relation to pregnancy, including keeping the baby, adoption, abortion and where to get further help

- Sexually transmitted infections (STIs)
- HIV/AIDs
- Safe sex
- STI screening, testing and treatments
- Alcohol and drugs and their impact on sex and relationships
- Puberty, male genitalia including the penis, scrotum, foreskin
- Male reproductive system, including testicles, urethra, semen, sperm and ejaculation
- Female genitalia, including vulva, labia minora and majora, clitoris, urethra and vaginal opening
- Female reproductive system, including uterus, ovaries, cervix and vagina
- The changing adolescent body, including discussion around pubic hair, wet dreams, masturbation and vaginal discharge
- The menstrual cycle
- Options for managing menstrual bleeding
- Self-examination, including testicular self-check, breast awareness and cervical screening

Once you have completed the activity, take a look at the topics which you feel most comfortable and confident to deliver. Ask yourself what the reason for this may be. Is it because these are areas you are most familiar with; do you have life experiences around these aspects which you can use to aid your practice? Is it because you have accessed prior training about the subject?

What about the topics which you found uncomfortable and where you lack the confidence to deliver them? Is this due to a lack of knowledge, skills and understanding, or linked to personal experiences which make the topic emotive or difficult for you? Could it be linked to your own values and beliefs?

Once you have identified these reasons, you can create a personal plan of action to address where you need to develop your skills and knowledge further.

Where you have a budget allocated, this could involve you booking onto and accessing some of the great training which is available. It could also involve a self-directed learning approach – you could read a book, or engage in online forums and groups. Another great way to develop your comfortableness is to shadow or work alongside a colleague.

Regardless of how much experience and confidence we have as a teacher or educator, talking about sex and relationships with young people is not always easy! Body parts, genitals, consent, periods and sex can be taboo subjects, many with stigma attached, which can make even the most experienced educators feel uncomfortable when they start to explore these new topics in the classroom with young people. And you can never know or fully prepare for what your students might say or ask. A fun activity to try to prepare for this is to create a list of possible questions students could ask in relation to the topic you will explore, and spend some time thinking about how you might respond to these. Resources like the FINK discussion cards can be helpful for this. How you will manage tricky questions is also an aspect which should be explored as part of your policy writing.

The final reflection activity is to think about your own personal relationships, sex and health education teaching philosophy and in one or two sentences, write down what you value as an RSE educator. It may require several adjustments before you decide who you are as a sex educator and your statement will evolve and develop as you grow into your role. Before writing my own, I asked a group of young people to draw a relationships and sex educator.

My relationship, sex and health education philosophy statement is as follows:

As an RSE educator, I believe that supporting the development of young people's critical thinking skills and developing them to become a confident and effective communicator is central to what I do. I am committed to providing teens with a safe space which allows them to explore their own values, get a grasp of new information, and create opportunities to practise their new skills.

Using realistic and relevant examples and thought-provoking questions, I encourage young people to know about and understand their own rights and responsibilities, which will help to keep themselves and each other safe.

I am passionate about making RSE fun, enjoyable and memorable and I do this by creating and planning workshops that include hands-on activities and interactive learning tools.

I work to build trusting and respectful relationships and role model the resilient, empowered and confident behaviours I want to see in the young people I educate. I do this by applying effective communication, having a genuine interest and passion for the subject and understanding and responding to their diverse needs.

◆ Chapter 3 ◆

Techniques for Teaching Sex Education

There is a range of different techniques included in the lesson activities within this resource. They are ones which have been specifically chosen to support the task or activity and to aid open and honest discussion through group work, paired working or reflective and independent working.

Before delivering your relationships and sex education programme, ground rules should be established with the group. Ground rules are a fundamental part of relationships and sex education and a key aspect when creating a safe space which will allow for open and honest discussion.

Establishing ground rules or a working agreement works best when you can involve the young people rather than just telling them what the rules are. Be mindful about allocating time at the beginning of the programme and also throughout to draw up a list of ground rules and revisit them when necessary. Consider where the rules or working agreement you create will be displayed and think about and agree with the young people what the consequences may be for anyone who does not follow them.

Some of the rules will be non-negotiable, for example a no mobile phone rule in your school or organization, or any other day-to-day classroom rules which will apply. You could also include statements about no racist, homophobic or sexist language, providing an opportunity to learn about the Equalities Act and its importance within RSE.

Respecting each other or respecting difference of opinions is often a ground rule shared by young people. But what exactly does respect mean to your group and in the context of this lesson, school or RSE?

Use the opportunity to talk to young people about how they would know if someone is being respectful. This discussion often leads to plenty more ideas for the ground rules list.

You should also use this opportunity to revisit and share with young people your school or organization's confidentiality policy and safeguarding procedures. Ensure that young people fully understand the consequences of sharing any personal information during discussion and activities and they know where they can go to access further support and help.

You could introduce a number of distancing techniques which young people could use to help them explore topics when sharing personal stories about themselves and others.

DISTANCING TECHNIQUES

Distancing techniques and activities are a quick and easy way for educators to de-personalize relationships and sex education topics that are being discussed. There are a number of ways you could do this; one way is to have the group create a few familiar characters that you can refer to in your discussion.

The group think of characters and then name them and give them a personality, deciding what they enjoy, their likes, dislikes, what they do and so on. The educator then uses the character to ask what they would do in this situation. How would they feel? What might they say? Other distancing techniques include using role play, or using characters from popular TV shows or real-life stories featured in news articles and magazines.

Tasking the young person to take on the role of a journalist or magazine writer, becoming a columnist and writing a problem page blog could also be used as a distancing tool for RSE.

Anonymous questions are great too. Provide opportunities for young people to submit their questions, online or via a post box. This is good for providing privacy for young people and it can also give you time to think more about your answers, helping you to manage any tricky questions you may receive.

Providing opportunities for open and honest conversation to take place is one of the most important aspects of RSE. In today's fast-moving, digital world, it is evident that young people can easily access many answers to any of the RSE-related questions they may have, but they often lack the opportunity to be able to sit, talk, debate, consider and share their ideas about health, relationships and sex education topics.

FACILITATING DISCUSSIONS

Group discussions require few tools and little equipment, which make them ideal for any working space or classroom environment. And when facilitated well, discussion activities can provide a safe and supportive environment for young people to practise talking about RSE topics, many which have huge stigma attached, which can help develop their own communication skills. Open and honest discussions, led by the teacher and managed well, can support young people to speak up, feeling safe enough to overcome any embarrassment they may have, and this can also lead to them feeling better about seeking health advice if and when they need it. Discussion activities do not have to be debates. Although debating is a great tool to use, be careful not to create a division within the class, particularly around topics which can be emotive such as abortion, sexual harassment or transgender issues.

If working with a large group, using a talking stick can be helpful. Anything can be used as the stick – a bean bag, marker pen, hairbrush. I use a squishy and stretchy stress toy shaped like an aubergine, which always goes down well in RSE. The tool itself leads to many great discussions.

If possible, you could also break larger groups into smaller working groups, allowing them a specific time to work on the task, before bringing the whole group back together at the end to summarize and share their learning experience with each other. Groups of around eight or more work best for effective discussions and allow a range of views to be heard.

Here are some suggestions for discussion activities you could introduce:

- *Talk stations:* Set posters up on the walls or on tables. Break the class into smaller groups and task them to travel from station to station in their groups. At each station, there should be some kind of task or prompt which will lead to the group having a conversation. They can also be encouraged to write down their answers and each group can read what the others have put and add to this.
- *This or that:* Read out loud a statement which has two possible responses, for example agree or disagree, yes or no, true or false. Depending on the young person's answer to the statement, they move to one side of the room or the other. From here, the young people can take turns and share the reasons for their answers and those with different ideas can also share their thoughts and views.
- *Backchannel:* A backchannel is a conversation that takes place alongside another activity. This is a communication method I often use at conferences or in my RSE teacher training. Share a video or read and present some information to young people and while this is happening, encourage the young people to use technology to submit their comments, suggestions, ideas and questions about what they are watching or listening to. There are many apps and websites you can use to allow this. I use Google Classroom, Slido or Canva. You could also incorporate this while delivering remote learning using the chat function, or broadcast live using social media and hashtags too.

When planning classroom discussions, think carefully about the question or statement you are going to introduce for the young people to discuss. Think openly about what the outcomes of this discussion could be. What further questions or topics might it lead to? How will you respond to these? How will you deal with any new concepts that are introduced which you didn't plan for and which you may not have the time to explore? One of my top tips for this is to set up an RSE display in the classroom which links to the topics you will cover that term. Here you can display key information which you may not have time to keep revisiting. You could also write a knowledge organizer, providing a summary of the key facts, diagrams and key terminology which you can hand out before or at the end of class. This can be a great tool for engaging parents.

Some young people may stay quiet during class discussions and so to involve them and capture their thoughts and opinions, you could provide them with a workbook. I am a big fan of workbooks and find them very useful, particularly in lessons which would ordinarily be presentation heavy. Use the workbook to provide a space where students can take notes, draw diagrams, complete quizzes and answer questions. Include reflective practice pages and learning logs, asking students to recap their group discussion, writing down their initial thoughts, what happened as part of the discussion and what they think and feel about the topic at the end.

And one final point: during discussions, don't forget to think about the classroom layout and how young people are sitting – if possible, allow the groups to move chairs or furniture and huddle together.

ROLE PLAY

Using drama and role play can support young people to safely practise new concepts and skills. A number of lessons in this resource use structured role play, which allocates time to planning and discussing the given scenario, demonstrating thoughts and ideas, and reaching a conclusion where the young people have the opportunity to discuss how they felt and what they learned. The most important part of role play is the reflection and discussion; costumes and props are not required but can be fun. I often use role play to explore topics such as healthy relationships, consent, safe sex and contraception. When role play is used as part of these lessons, the young people are able to practise their communication skills in a safe, non-threatening environment, consider different perspectives and develop empathy by seeing how their decisions might affect others and solve social problems.

PROBLEM-SOLVING

As young people grow up and navigate their teens, they will encounter many situations in which they will need to make important life decisions. When young people have been given the opportunity to solve problems themselves in a safe classroom environment, they develop the confidence and skills that will enable them to do this in other aspects of their lives. This book uses real-life and relevant situations which are then explored through the use of guided questions. These conversations prompt reflection, questioning and modelling, and can provide new and useful language and terminology.

◆ Chapter 4 ◆

Language and Terminology

One of the biggest barriers that prevents educators from delivering open and honest relationships and sex education is the language which is connected to it. As part of your lessons, you will use a range of language including the correct terminology, medical and scientific words, as well as street slang or jargon. It may be useful, as part of your reflection activities and preparation, to identify any words or terms which you feel uncomfortable with and unpick the connotation behind these to help you understand the reasons for your feelings. It can also be very useful to practise in advance what you are going to say and have a go at saying it out loud, by yourself and in front of others.

Language, particularly the words spoken in RSE, can be funny and often leads to fits of giggles, especially if the group are not used to hearing such words. Consider what the reactions to the terminology you use may be and think about how you might deal with this in advance. It would be best not to remove a young person from a lesson because they find it funny, so strategies that develop a comfortableness will be useful. One way to introduce the use of sex education language and terminology – which I use all the time in my workshops and training – is an icebreaker called The A–Z of Sex Ed. This can be done individually, in teams or as a whole class. The goal is to find a word associated with sex education for each letter of the alphabet. It is important to let the group know in advance that any word is acceptable, including both slang words and correct terminology, but also use this opportunity to revisit the ground rules and explain that any sexist or homophobic language is unacceptable. Let the young people know that any term they are unsure of they can ask or write down. This provides a great opportunity for open discussion about language which young people may have heard but don't fully understand. The activity often leads to lots of laughter, but it can also be a great tool to help you identify where the group are at and what they have already been exposed to. For example, in one of my groups, this activity prompted great discussion which started from a particular word but led to the challenging of sexist views which had been reinforced by porn.

When reading through the A–Z list with the group, you can provide the correct terminology for any slang words used. For example, if a group have written 'BJs', I would use this opportunity to say that we will be using the term oral sex as part of our RSE learning. You may also come across new terms which you have not heard of. Make a note of these, brace yourself and check the definition online at Urban Dictionary. Another simple way to introduce language and overcome any barriers is to create knowledge organizers linked to your topic and include key terms and descriptions. You can also display these in the classroom.

NON-JUDGEMENTAL AND INCLUSIVE LANGUAGE

When delivering RSE we should never assume to know a person's sexuality, sexual preferences or experiences. I remember seeing a lesson being delivered where the teacher said, 'I know that all young people your age sext', and another where the teacher stated, 'When you are older and have a wife...' These assumptions can be harmful and can prevent young people from engaging in the learning and assume that the information is not for them. So, considering your choice of language is very important. Use language which is less prescriptive and more inclusive to all. An example of this is using the term partner in place of husband/wife, girlfriend/boyfriend. Another example is saying, 'if you *chose* to send a sext', rather than, '*when* you send a sext', which reinforces the idea that this is something that all young people do. Be mindful of reinforcing sexist stereotypes such as referring to doctors as male and nurses as female. When we think carefully about the language we use we can support more young people to feel included.

◆ Chapter 5 ◆

Sex Education Pathway or Timeline

There is so much talk about what is age-appropriate and which topics should be introduced at which age and why. And the answer to this is that there is no one size fits all answer. What is age-appropriate for one group may be too little or too much for another and so understanding the needs of your communities and students is another important aspect of relationships, sex and health education.

We do know that topics are best introduced before young people have experienced them. This gives young people the knowledge and skills to be able to make better informed choices. So, when planning for RSE, we should always aim to be proactive and prepare young people for the social dilemmas and situations ahead.

It can be helpful to learn more about the local area where you are delivering your work. Which communities does your school or organization serve and what are the issues facing these communities on a local scale? Things such as high teenage conception rates and sexually transmitted infections among the under 25s can be relevant. If you create a local RSE network, you will be able to obtain an up-to-date and relevant picture of your local area and the people living in it, and prepare a curriculum in response to this.

Also consider national guidance and data, such as that provided by government, the Office for National Statistics, lesbian, gay, bisexual, transgender, queer or questioning, intersex and asexual (LGBTQIA+) organizations, and charities that support victims of relationship violence and abuse. Figures released by the Office for National Statistics show that in 2019 there were 212,000 same-sex families in the UK, which helps us recognize the need for diverse families to feature within our RSE delivery.

You should also consider any additional learning requirements of students and plan for this accordingly. The government has made clear in its guidance that all young people are entitled to relationships, sex and health education, including those with special educational needs and disabilities. Consider how you can adapt resources and materials to ensure that all students can take part.

When developing your RSE curriculum, it can help to create and plan a learning pathway to support the learning process and help set RSE priorities, identifying the key topics that you will need more time and space to elaborate on and maybe revisit each year, and other subjects that may be covered only once. It can be helpful to develop the RSE pathway in close coordination with other education programme plans such as ICT and safeguarding initiatives, to see where there may be crossover or opportunities to revisit and build on pre-existing knowledge.

Have a go at creating your own RSE learning timeline. This activity could be carried out by educators, parents and young people, comparing the answers. It is a great tool to guide curriculum planning.

First, create a timeline, starting from Year 7 to Year 11 for secondary school-aged young people. Next, compile a range of topic cards – you could use the RSE guidance learning outcomes to create these. Using the cards, ask participants to place the card on the timeline at the stage they think the topic should be explored and taught. Discuss what the reasons are for this choice and in what circumstances they would consider introducing the topic earlier or later.

| YEAR 7 | YEAR 8 | YEAR 9 | YEAR 10 | YEAR 11 |

YEAR 7

A transition programme for Year 6 pupils in partnership with feeder primary schools: developing self-esteem, communication skills and decision-making. Health education covering puberty and periods. Bullying and online safety, friendships, relationships, boundaries and consent. Gender stereotypes, FGM, getting help and helping others.

YEAR 8

Values, peer pressure, respectful relationships, and personal safety. Laws around sexting, and how to deal with harmful content online. What is grooming? Understanding how to spot and report child sexual exploitation.

YEAR 9

What does an unhealthy relationship look like? How does the media impact you? What is consent? Is everybody doing it? Get to know your body, learn about sexually transmitted infections. Develop the skills and knowledge to negotiate boundaries in friendships and relationships and have an open and honest chat about safer sex.

YEAR 10

What actually is sexual harassment, upskirting and victim-blaming? Should we really worry about the impact of porn on teens? What are your contraceptive choices? Learning the skills needed to carry out testicular self-examination (TSE) and breast self-examination (BSE).

YEAR 11

How do you access health care, and what do you need to know about your body and fertility to live a healthy and happy life? Where do you get STI screening? Living with HIV. What is forced marriage? Revenge porn? And online dating? How can you recognize and get help with abusive relationships?

To support the development of young people's knowledge, skills and attitudes it can be helpful to map out the learning pathway young people will take. The pathway highlights the framework for learning for each year group. The progression model will help you revisit and build on the learning of key topics. I include in the pathway any transition plans and partnerships to ensure I bridge any gaps in RSE from primary school to secondary school.

Part 2

RESOURCES FOR DELIVERING RELATIONSHIPS, SEX AND HEALTH EDUCATION

This book provides activities and ideas to explore and discuss relationships, sex and health education topics with young people. The resource features workshop activity ideas and suggested discussion points which can aid your delivery in a classroom or group work setting, as well as worksheets and handouts. Where the resources are downloadable, a symbol has been added to indicate this. These pages can be downloaded from https://library.jkp.com/redeem using the code FJFQVCH.

The activities will provide you with a starting point and allow you to open up and have conversations with young people.

The book is designed to be flexible, and so no timings have been included. This is to encourage you to adapt and adjust the activities to meet the different spaces, timing, ages and stages of the young people. The activities are ones that I have used many times with young people, and over the past 25 years they have been tweaked in response to the changing world and the feedback from young people, teachers and parents. The activities are great for RSE, large groups and small groups and also work well for youth work and informal education settings.

Find your own style of delivery, make the sessions your own, have confidence in what you do and recognize the importance of the messages you will teach. Don't forget that the best and most effective relationships and sex education resource is you.

◆ Chapter 6 ◆

Relationships Education

INTRODUCTION

Teachers, teaching assistants, youth workers and other professionals working with children and young people play an important role in supporting the development of healthy relationships skills.

The aim of relationships education is to provide students with the knowledge and skills they need to help them form healthy and respectful friendships and romantic relationships. It works best when it leads on from primary school learning that incorporates lessons about family and friendships.

To equip young people with the skills they need for life in modern Britain, it is vital that your curriculum reflects the full diversity of the world in which we live and so it is important to ensure that same-sex and heterosexual relationships, people with disabilities and people of different faiths, cultures and colour are included within your lessons about relationships.

Your curriculum framework, lesson plans and activities should aim to provide learning opportunities which enable young people to know what a healthy relationship looks like and what makes a good friend, a good work colleague and a husband, wife or life partner. Lessons which explore acceptable and unacceptable behaviour in relationships should also be included, supporting young people to recognize how unhealthy relationships can impact their mental wellbeing, and how to manage these situations and access support if they need it.

According to the United Nations Convention on the Rights of the Child (1989), one of the most basic human rights principles is the right to live free from the threat of violence. We know that young people are one of the vulnerable groups most likely to be in an abusive relationship. A recent survey of 13–17-year-olds highlighted in the *Not Just Collateral Damage* report from Barnardo's (James 2020) that a quarter (25 per cent) of girls and 18 per cent of boys reported having experienced some form of physical violence from an intimate partner.

Another report from Women's Aid in partnership with Avon (2015), which spoke to young women aged 16–24 years, found that only one in three women understood what coercive control meant, and one in 20 young women assumed that being scared of their partner was a normal and acceptable part of relationships.

We also now know that many LGBTQIA+ young people do not feel represented in RSE lessons and that LGBTQIA+ bullying is common throughout primary schools, so it's essential that young people are provided with the opportunities to develop inclusive attitudes. The Equality Act 2010 lists 'gender reassignment' and 'sexual orientation' as protected characteristics, as well as disability and religion or belief, meaning that all schools have a duty to make sure that their students are not discriminated against, either because of their faith and/or because they are LGBTQIA+.

FRIENDS

Introducing the topic: Having a friend that you like spending time with and can trust is an important aspect of growing up. It feels amazing when two friends show kindness and care and support each other. But what is it that makes someone a good friend? And how can we better deal with life situations which may cause friends to argue and sometimes even fall out?

ACTIVITY: BEING A GOOD FRIEND

Work with young people to explore their thoughts around what it takes to be a good friend. Give them examples of friendship characteristics and ask them if they can think of more of their own.

▼ Friendship characteristics

Trustworthy	Loyal	Non-judgemental	Likes my family
Honest	Caring	Similar interest	Helpful
Good listener	Attentive	Respects me	Same age as me
Supportive	Fun	Empathizes	Funny
Forgiving	Generous	Confident	Dependable

Friendships can be developed within families, in school, within groups and even over the internet. But being a good friend is not a skill that everybody just has.

Developing friendships skills can take lots of work. One way to develop friendship skills is to ask the young people to recognize which of the friendship characteristics listed they have, and to think about how a friend would describe them.

Extend the activity by tasking the young people to write down ten 'I am' statements which describe them as a friend. For example:

1. I am honest.
2. I am supportive.

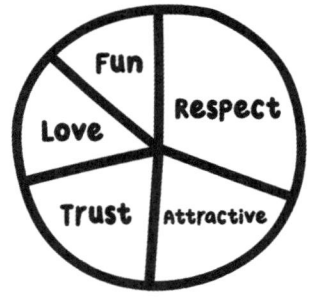

Using the list of important friendship characteristics provided and the ones from the young people's own list, task the group to make a good friendship pie chart. This is a visual tool which can help young people explore their relationship personal values. It should be based on all the friendship qualities that are most important to them. Remind them to give a higher percentage to the attributes which are more important.

TALKING POINTS

- Are there different types of friend? If so, what are they?
- What makes a good friend?
- What qualities would a good friend have?
- What would a best friend be like?
- What about 'online' friends? Are they different from the friends you make in real life, at school or at home?

Sometimes friendships can become stressful, people can change and develop new interests and hobbies and make new friendship groups. It can be sad when this happens.

Ask the young people to share their thoughts and state what advice they would give to someone who was in this situation. Explain where young people can go in school and the local community to get further advice and information about making friends, friendships and falling out.

ROMANCE AND LOVE

Introducing the topic: Developing romantic feelings for another person is totally normal. It's also totally normal if you do not experience romantic relationships. But how do you know if you are in love? And what actually is romance?

Start the session off with a quick group activity. Breaking the young people into small groups, task them to think about and write down answers to these key questions:

- What does the word relationship mean?
- What different types of relationship are there?
- What are the positives about relationships?
- What are the negatives about relationships?

Facilitate the young people to share their responses with other groups. Did they have similar ideas? To develop their understanding further, work together as a whole group to create a group/class definition for the term 'Relationship'.

The topic has a number of activities which you can use with young people to look at love and romance further. Choose one of more, depending on how much time you have.

ACTIVITY: IF LOVE WAS A...

The word 'love' can be used to explain how we feel about people – romantically, in friendships, as relatives – but we also use it when we talk fondly about the things that we like, such as food that we love or sports and music. Reflecting on what love feels and looks like can help us to know when our relationships are good and healthy and when they may be negative or unhealthy.

Using a dictionary, look up and read through the different definitions of love.

For the activity, ask the young people to use the sentence starters to write their ideas about what love feels like:

If love was a sound, it would be: . . . .

If love was a texture, it would be: . . . .

If love was a smell, it would be: . . . .

If love was a taste, it would be: . . . .

If love was a colour, it would be: . . . .

If love was a place, it would be: . . . .

If love was a song, it would be: . . . .

If love was a person, it would be: . . . .

If love was the weather, it would be: . . . .

ACTIVITY: THE LOVE SONG PLAYLIST

Create a playlist of love songs with the young people which focus on love within a romantic relationship. Listen to the songs and interpret what the lyrics say about love, romance and relationships.

ACTIVITY: IS THIS A ROMANTIC RELATIONSHIP?

Start a discussion with the young people about what the following terms mean in today's society.

Going out with, sleeping together, in love, having sex, making love, making out (add any more which are relevant to your group and communities).

Do these terms imply that the people involved are in a romantic relationship?

Being in a romantic relationship or being in love doesn't mean you have to have an intimate or sexual relationship. Discuss other ways that people who are in love can show they are attracted to and care for another person. For example, holding hands, having loving conversations, enjoying cuddles, sitting on a knee, being held, lying together, doing fun hobbies together, laughing together, touching (non-sexual), eating together, dancing.

DIGITAL DATING

Introducing the topic: Online relationships can have different purposes. They can be friendships, where you chat about day-to-day things and similar interests and just hang out; support groups where you are sharing with others who may be going through similar experiences to you; networks where you might be learning from others and developing new skills; and also dating, where you develop a romantic relationship with a person online, which could also lead to meeting in person.

Dating people digitally has become more popular in recent years, as the internet and social media apps offer many new ways for people to meet and talk to others. Even though it is fun and exciting to talk to and develop loving and caring relationships with people online, it is also important to learn about some of the risks involved in digital dating.

ACTIVITY: THE DOS AND DON'TS OF DIGITAL DATING

Ask the young people if they have heard of any online dating apps. Do they know the age restrictions for these? Do people who have relationships online only date via these apps? What about relationships which develop on other social media platforms or websites – can this be digital dating too?

Ask the young people to create a table which shows the positives and negatives of digital dating (or making friends online). They can do this as a whole-group activity using the whiteboard or some large paper, or work in pairs or small groups.

If working in smaller groups, bring all the answers together to create one table that features ideas from everybody. From the answers suggested, explore further the potential dangers young people may face through digital dating.

Some of the answers listed may include:

- Risk of grooming
- Consequences of sexting
- Privacy concerns
- Online bullying or harassment.

What can young people do to reduce these risks?

Encourage discussion with young people around solutions which can help them reduce their risk when developing friendships and relationships online. Some suggestions are listed below:

Grooming – understand what the signs to look out for are, and know how to report and seek help if they think this may be happening to them.

Sexting – understand they have the right to say no, and know the laws around sexting.

Privacy – know how to manage settings on apps and websites, understand why it is important not to share personal information.

Online bullying/harassment – know how to report and have the resilience skills to cope with any negative comments, unwelcome advances and sexually explicit pictures.

ACTIVITY: BLOG POSTS

A great way to conclude the session and to capture what young people have learned about the topic is to ask them to choose one of the risks of digital dating, and write a blog post aimed at young people which will help them to understand the risks associated with online dating and relationships.

They must remember to include some top tips sharing some of the ways to stay safe online. Also important to mention are links to local or national support organizations where a young person reading the blog could go for help if they needed it.

SEXTING

Introducing the topic: More and more young people now use technology, smartphones and social media to communicate in their relationships. Many use these methods to connect with people they know in person, like mums, dads, cousins and friends. Online is also a space where people make new friends too. And just like in real life, we have to be mindful of our online behaviours and ensure that we treat people online with the same respect we would if we met them face to face.

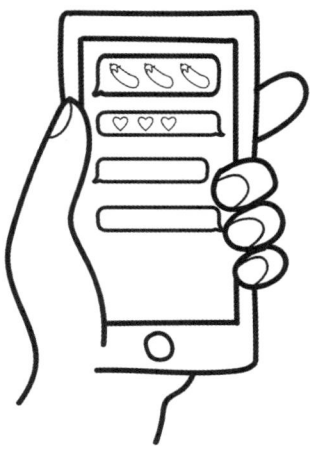

In England and across the world, there are specific laws which relate to our online behaviours and how we use technology.

Sexting is one of these online behaviours which can have a legal consequence.

WHAT IS SEXTING?

Sexting is when sexual photographs, videos or messages are sent to friends, romantic partners or strangers online. Sexting can include sending or sharing images and videos where the person is partly or fully naked; sometimes people call these 'nudes'.

Sexting includes sending, receiving or sharing sexually explicit text messages, emails and voice notes. It also covers any sexual acts which are posted on a live stream, webcam or video call.

The law states that anyone who has or sends indecent images of someone under the age of 18 is breaking the law. Storing and distributing sexual images is also an offence under the Sexual Offences Act (2003, 2021). Encouraging someone to take or send 'sexts' can also be illegal.

ACTIVITY: LET'S TALK ABOUT SEXT

Use the talking points, information and guidance below, encourage a discussion with young people about sexting laws and young people's online, digital behaviours around sexting.

Despite knowing the laws and risks associated with sexting, some young people still sext. Many think it is the normal thing to do and that everybody is doing it. Write the following sentence on the board, giving each young person a sticky note to write their suggested answer.

One in . . . . young people aged 14 and over say they have sent a sext.

According to the 2020 report *Look At Me: Teens, Sexting and Risks* (Katz & El Asam 2020), one in six young people say they have sent an image of themselves to someone else.

Explore some of the other reasons that young people sext.

For some teens, sexting is a fun way to explore their sexuality. Others have said that sharing images makes them feel happier about their bodies and the attention they receive makes them feel confident.

Some people also say that they have sent sexts after being pressured. This is worrying. Sexting should be consensual between people over the age of 18.

Here is what pressure to send a sext can look like:

- Worrying that you won't be liked or the relationship will end if you don't.
- Being asked again and again, not having boundaries respected.
- Being made to feel guilty.
- Being called names to add pressure, such as 'cold' or 'frigid'.
- Receiving or being offered gifts.

Ask the young people what advice they would give to a young person who said they were feeling pressured to sext.

ACTIVITY: SEXTING LAWS LEAFLET FOR TEENS

Task the young people, in groups or pairs, to create a leaflet for teens which highlights the sexting laws, and can make them aware of what pressure to sext looks like. Remember that it should include details of where to get further advice or support.

SEXUALITY

Introducing the topic: Sexuality is about how people experience sexual and romantic attraction. It includes a person's interest and preferences around sexual and romantic relationships and may include the way they identify themselves. Sexuality can be fluid, which means it can change.

Sex, gender reassignment and sexuality are protected characteristics in the Equalities Act 2010. This means it is against the law to discriminate against someone because of these things. Watch a video from YouTube which explains more about the Equalities Act and protected characteristics. Take a look at The Equality and Human Rights Commission, which is Great Britain's national equality body.

Understanding the language that describes different types of sexual and romantic feelings and orientations can help all of us to be more respectful of the diverse world in which we live.

ACTIVITY: SEXUALITY DEFINITION SORTING CARDS

 Download, print and cut out the sexuality definition cards. Mix them up and use these cards to see if the young people can match the sexuality term to the correct definition.

Asexual	A term describing individuals who don't experience sexual attraction to others of any gender.
Bisexual	A sexual orientation that describes those who experience sexual, romantic or emotional attractions to people of more than one gender.
Coming out	The process of being open about your sexuality and gender.
Fluid	This term refers to the fact that sexuality, sexual attraction and sexual behaviour can change over time.
Gay	A term that describes a man or male-identified person who has sexual, romantic or emotional attraction to people of the same gender.
Heterosexual	A word which describes people who experience sexual, romantic or emotional attraction to people of the opposite gender (e.g. male and female).

Lesbian	A woman or female-identified person who experiences sexual, romantic or emotional attraction to people of the same or a similar gender.
LGBTQIA+	An acronym for lesbian, gay, bisexual, transgender, queer or questioning, intersex and asexual.
Pansexual	A term that describes individuals who can experience sexual, romantic or emotional attraction to any person, regardless of that person's gender, sex or sexuality.
Questioning	The process of being curious about or exploring some aspect of sexuality or gender.

TALKING POINTS

Use these prompts to conclude the sexuality definition card activity:

- Do you have any further questions about sexuality?
- How can we ensure that young people in our group/school or community feel welcome and accepted?
- What can we do about any discrimination?

CELEBRATING DIVERSITY

Many schools and organizations celebrate and host events linked to diversity days. Here are some suggestions:

- Hold a fashion show to celebrate traditional clothing from around the world.
- Organize a sporting event related to a national campaign such as Rainbow Laces Day.
- Arrange a Pride parade or get involved in your local one.
- Get young people to create rainbows or campaign materials.

GENDER STEREOTYPES

Introducing the topic: Our understanding and ideas about gender roles and gender norms come from a variety of places, they can be developed from the perceptions we have learned from families, or picked up from key messages we see in the media, they may grow from our own ideas based on our life experiences and from what we see in our communities, or in wider society.

From childhood, we develop our understanding of gender roles which we then use to make our choices about what things (places, jobs, colours, clothes, hobbies, interests, language, hair, personalities and behaviours) are associated with being male or female. Many people then conform to these roles and identify with them.

THE GENDERBREAD PERSON

The Genderbread Person (see the Resources section) is a teaching tool for breaking the big concept of gender down into bite-sized, digestible pieces. Using posters and worksheets, it unpicks the concepts of gender into a number of different aspects: sex, gender identity, gender expression. Sexual orientation is also included due to its close connection to gender identity and expression.

Discuss:

- Why is understanding about gender stereotypes important?
- What impact do you think stereotypes about gender can have on relationships?

Gender roles and stereotyping have been proven to influence our behaviours and relationships. They can lead to a misinformed idea of relationship roles and expectations that reinforce the idea of gender-specific behaviours, which can be harmful.

Following these gender roles and norms can lead to a young person engaging with risky behaviour. An example of this is around boys and masculinity; following the stereotypes of what it means to be a man can lead to young men being less likely to show emotion or to seek help when they need it. They may be more aggressive and deal with conflict in a violent way rather than talking it out.

Providing learning opportunities and safe spaces for young people to explore gender equality and the effects of gender stereotypes could help to prevent relationship violence and abuse. Although relationship violence and abuse can happen to anyone of any age, gender or sexual orientation, the vast majority of relationship abuse happens to women and the perpetrators are most often men. Many studies have highlighted a clear and definite link between men who have committed crimes against their female partners and misogynistic beliefs. To tackle and reduce incidences of relationship abuse and to allow young people to better understand respectful relationships, equality and topics including sexism should be introduced, alongside any sexist or discriminatory comments or behaviour being challenged.

Activities which involve exploring attitudes, beliefs and values are an important aspect of relationships, sex and health education.

ACTIVITY: GENDER BINARY

Facilitate this activity for young people. It works better when young people have the space to stand up and move around but can be adapted if this is not an option.

After creating a large open space for moving, begin by asking all young people to stand in the middle of the room. The right side of the room represents the answer 'girl/female/women' and the left side 'boy/male/men'. This introductory activity is a fun way to begin to explore this topic about gender stereotypes, but remember to revisit the ground rules you developed before beginning RSE, particularly any which say we should be non-judgemental, listen to each other and challenge any comments we disagree with respectfully.

Ask the young people to listen carefully to the following words which will be read out (and/or displayed on the board if space to move around is not available). The young people should move to the side of the room which they feel the word is better or more associated with:

Hero	Dance	Teacher	Aggressive
Cooking	Pink	Cars	Doctor
Loving	Fit	Scientist	Cleaner
Solicitor	Tool box	Gamer	Glitter
Make-up artist	Emotional	Face creams	Farting and burping

After the activity explore the findings with the group.

- Did they mostly agree or was there a clear divide?
- Where do they think their answers and ideas about these 'choices' or 'assumptions' come from?

Ask the young people to reflect on whether we absolutely fit into the gender roles and ideas which are associated with being male or female.

ACTIVITY: GENDER STEREOTYPE STATEMENT CARDS

Break young people into small groups and provide each with a copy of the gender stereotype statement cards. The young people should read the statement cards which have a common stereotype written on them and consider how these ways of thinking can negatively impact on respectful and healthy relationships. Ask them what can be done to challenge these ideas.

Boys will be boys.	Men are not great when talking about their feelings.
When a boy pushes or teases you, it's because he really likes you.	All girls want to grow up, get married and have a baby.
It is a women's responsibility to plan for contraceptive use.	Men who have had lots of sexual partners are really cool.
It is a man's responsibility to plan the use of condoms.	Women who have had lots of sexual partners are promiscuous.
Real men don't cry.	Girls say 'no' to sex at first to try and look more respectful.
Stop crying like a girl.	Most boys are only after one thing.
Men should be the ones to initiate sex.	Man up.

SEXISM

◆

Introducing the topic: Sexist messages in popular culture and the media often reinforce gender and sexist stereotypes. In June 2019 following a review of gender stereotyping in advertising, the Advertising Standards Authority put a ban of any adverts that reinforce 'harmful' stereotypes that can restrict people's choices and opportunities.

ACTIVITY: RE-WRITE THE AD

Collect a number of examples of sexist adverts which depict gender stereotypes. These could be print advertisements, radio or video. Some good examples which have worked well with groups include the 'Bic for Her' pens, available in a variety of pretty pastel shades such as lavender and mint. They were described in the advertising as having an 'elegant design, just for her!' and a 'thin barrel to fit a women's hand'.

The People Per Hour London underground advert 'You do the girl boss thing. We'll do the SEO thing' was banned by the Advertising Standards Authority (2020) which concluded that it implied that women were not skilled at using technology.

Another great example, which stereotypes men, was the 2019 TV advert and video on demand (VOD) ad for the soft cheese, Philadelphia by Mondelez UK Ltd. This received complaints saying that the advert perpetuated a harmful stereotype of men by suggesting they were incapable of caring for children.

Research the adverts, looking at what happened: what was the outcry and backlash, how did they make certain groups feel, what was the outcome? With the young people working in pairs or small groups ask them to choose and re-create an advert, correcting the sexism. They could re-write the script, or get creative and use role play or digital design.

RESPECTFUL RELATIONSHIPS

Introducing the topic: If and when a young person decides they want to be in a relationship with someone, it is important that they understand and are able to recognize the differences between a respectful relationship and any signs which would suggest a relationship is becoming unhealthy.

A few important qualities of a respectful relationship are good communication, relationships built on trust and a partnership where both people's feelings and boundaries are respected. Young people will most likely have some of their own ideas about what qualities are important for respectful relationships too.

Respect is one of the qualities that is often mentioned when thinking about the important ingredients that make up a healthy relationship. But respect can mean different things to different people.

ACTIVITY: 100 PER CENT MY TYPE ON PAPER

This fun drawing task was made popular by the TV programme *Love Island*. It involved contestants being asked to draw and write down what they would describe as '100 per cent my type on paper', which is another way of saying their ideal partner.

 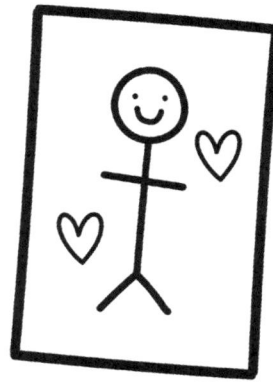

For this task, the young people are asked to draw and also write down or list any key words which describe what their ideal 'long-term or lifelong' partner would be like. Encourage them to think of at least 10–15 points. They should think about the kind of traits (behaviours, characteristics, personality) and qualities (abilities, talents) and anything else that are important to their relationships.

For ideas, see the list of words collected from other young people's list and drawings.

▼ 100 per cent my type on paper – word list

Caring	Loyal	Strong	Pretty	Handsome
Respectful	Good listener	Easy to talk to	Empathizes	Tall
Small	Loving	Caring	Kind	Funny
Happy	Emotional	Healthy	Fit	Energetic
Relaxed	Has similar interests	Likes my family	Mutual friends	Independent
Reliable	Honest	Compliments me	Confident	Extroverted
Introverted	Uses social media	Is my age	Faithful	Sensitive
Aggressive	Assertive	Passive	Has money	Fashionable
Good hygiene	Buys me gifts	Has time for me	Committed	Successful

TALKING POINTS

Use these questions to prompt further discussion:

- What are some examples of the characteristics you have listed or drawn?
- Are there many similarities, or major differences?
- Where do these ideas about what would make the 'ideal partner' come from?
- Do you spot any stereotypical roles or behaviours in your list or drawings (breadwinner, strong, caring, kind)?
- Where do you think young people see respectful relationship behaviours and traits being modelled?
- How does the media represent teens and romantic relationships?
- Thinking about your ideal partner drawing and list, can you identify the key points or things which are 100 per cent required and those which are negotiable and where you may compromise?

ACTIVITY: VOX POP

A vox pop is often used in the media, in news and radio, to provide a snapshot of public opinion. Short for Latin *vox populi* meaning 'voice of the people', a vox pop is where lots of different people are approached and are asked to give their views on a particular topic. Their responses are then presented to showcase what is the most popular opinion.

Task the young people with using a recording device (voice notes on smartphones would do) to create their own respectful relationships vox pop. These are the steps they will have to bear in mind:

1. Set up the recording device.
2. Practise interviewing and recording with a partner.
3. Choose a key question: some example vox pop questions could be: What does the word 'respect' mean in a romantic relationship? Describe how respect is show in a relationship?
4. Decide who the questions will be aimed at: identify a variety of people, ages, backgrounds and so on.
5. Ask the questions and record the answers.
6. Edit the vox pop.
7. Share the vox pops with the rest of the groups.

Discuss with the young people what the most popular opinion was. What did they learn from listening to all the different ideas about respect in relationships?

If the young people don't have access to recording devices, they could print copies of speech bubbles and get people to write their answers inside these instead. You could use these to create a display.

ACTIVITY: RESPECT DISCUSSION STARTERS

Split young people into three groups and task each group with a discussion starter activity. Allow the young people time to explore and discuss the topic area and carry out the suggested activity.

⊙ Discussion starters

Respecting diversity: No two people are ever the same – and being different is something that we should celebrate. There are some differences that can result in people being discriminated against. People from different cultural backgrounds, people in a same-sex relationship, people living with a disability are just some of the groups who experience discrimination based on their differences. Being respectful of diversity means being inclusive, celebrating difference, and making sure that everyone's voice is heard. What do the terms tolerance and empowerment mean and why are they important to respecting diversity? Using a dictionary read the definitions of respect, diversity, tolerance and empowerment. Can you rewrite the meaning of the worlds into sentences which are more designed for young people?

Respect online: Respect in relationships is just as important online as it is in person. How can young people show respect online? There are laws in place which link to online behaviours and how we use technology respectfully. Can you name any of these laws? Have a look at the Equality Act 2010, the Communications Act 2003, the Protection from Harassment Act 1997, and the Malicious Communications Act 1988. What do they say which links to respect online?

Boundaries and privacy: In a healthy relationship, both partners are entitled to have their own boundaries and privacy respected. Consider and explore the idea that respect within a romantic relationship is about sharing account passwords, and giving up your own privacy. For some young people, this may mean sharing or giving a partner access to their social media accounts.

ACTIVITY: RESPECTFULLY DISAGREE

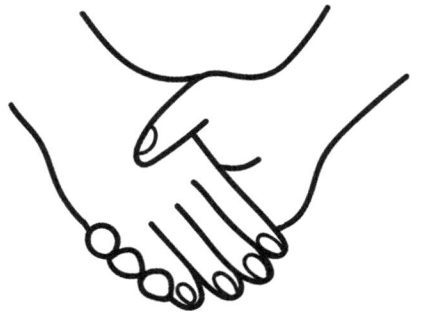

No relationship is ever perfect and there will almost definitely be moments in romantic relationships when minor disagreements will happen. This activity will allow us to practice skills to respectfully disagree and can be carried out as a whole group or in smaller groups, with each group given a few topics to explore.

Download, print and cut out the topic cards. Place them in the middle of the group. Each person takes a statement and reads it out loud. They share their view about the topic on the card with the rest of their group including the reasons why they think this way. Other members of the group are invited to share their thoughts too. They may agree with the person's comments and can say they do, also explaining why. Some young people may disagree, and they can also be encouraged to share the reasons why they think differently. Facilitate and manage the discussion respectfully, allowing people to listen to each other, share opinions, and, where needed, agree to disagree. Refer back where necessary to the working agreement/ground rules established at the beginning of the RSE work.

▼ Discussion cards

Monogamy	Cheating in a relationship	Casual hook-ups	Dating apps	Abstinence
Teen relationship abuse	Sharing social media passwords with partner	Checking your partner's text messages	Dating someone older	Compulsory sex education
Sex to have a baby	Sex for pleasure	Contraceptive choices	Free condoms for under 25s	Paying for emergency contraception

LAWS ABOUT BEING RESPECTFUL ONLINE

These are some of the laws that apply to behaviour online.

Equality Act 2010: This supports the notion that everyone has the right to be treated with dignity and respect. The Equality Act forbids discrimination against any person based on any of the protected characteristics: age, disability, gender, pregnancy and maternity, race, religion or belief, sex and sexual orientation.

Communications Act 2003: This covers various different communications. Some of the issues the act protects against are threatening behaviour online and offensive and indecent images.

Protection from Harassment Act 1997: Harassment is when someone behaves in a way which makes you feel distressed, humiliated or threatened. Examples of harassment include unwanted phone calls, letters, emails and abuse and bullying online. Harassment is both a criminal offence and a civil action.

Malicious Communications Act 1988: This makes it illegal in England and Wales to 'send or deliver letters or other articles for the purpose of causing distress or anxiety'. It also applies to electronic communications.

Search for respect campaigns and share some positive examples, such as the Football Association's Respect Programme, Kick it Out and the Union of European Football Associations' (UEFA) EqualGame. These campaigns are used to promote respect, tolerance and to empower communities through sport.

PEER PRESSURE

Introducing the topic:

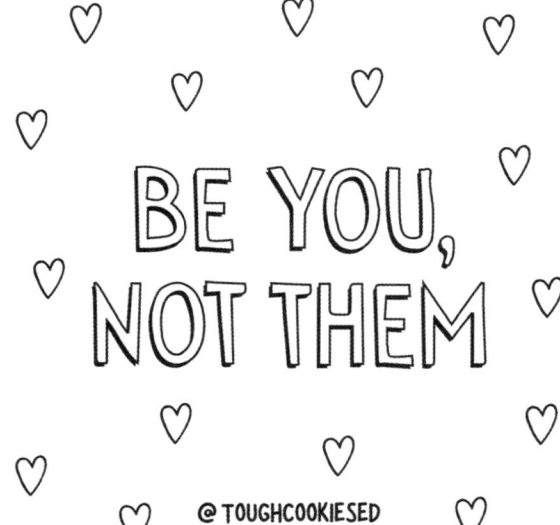

- What is a peer/s?
  A peer is a person or group of people who have similar interests, age and background. They can be a friend, neighbour, family member or just someone you know.

- What is pressure?
  Pressure in this context is feeling as if you have to do something.

- What is peer pressure?
  Peer pressure is when your friends or peers try to persuade or pressure you to do something. Peer pressure can be positive or negative.

- What is an example of positive peer pressure?
  Peer pressure can be positive if the encouragement gets you to do something you didn't want to do, for example if you were nervous to join a new dance class and your peers pressured you into going, you might overcome your fears and do something good.

- What kind of situations might involve negative peer pressure?
  Negative peer pressure could include the pressure to act or behave in a certain manner, such as to skip class, stay out later than you are allowed, run away from home, or take something that is not yours. There can be a pressure to look a certain way or to wear certain clothes. It could involve the pressure to take risks, like smoking cigarettes, drinking alcohol and even engaging in sexual activity before you feel ready to.

ACTIVITY: WHAT DOES PEER PRESSURE SOUND LIKE, LOOK LIKE AND FEEL LIKE TO YOU?

Ask the young people to draw, write or describe what peer pressure looks like, sounds like and feels like to them. When they understand this better, it can help them to notice when it is happening.

Look	Sound	Feel

ACTIVITY: WHAT WOULD YOU DO?

To help deal with peer pressure, ask the young people to think about some of the possible situations they could experience and to prepare an exit plan. An exit plan is an idea of what someone might say or do if they found themselves in a situation. Here is an example of an exit plan.

Sam was going to a sleepover with a group of friends. Later in the evening people at the sleepover had started to experiment with drugs and some members of the group who Sam didn't know that well were putting pressure on her to do the same. Sam texted a house emoji to her parents. When they received the text, they immediately called Sam and said family emergency, and she needed to come home. This was a plan Sam had agreed beforehand to help deal with any uncomfortable situations.

What exit plans could be put in place to help young people who were being pressured to:

- vape
- bully someone on public transport
- have a beauty treatment (such as waxing)
- send a nude image
- smash a window?

ACTIVITY: COMMUNICATING BOUNDARIES

Boundaries are the limits and rules that people set for themselves in relationships. Practising how to share your thoughts in an honest but respectful way is healthier than avoiding any awkward situations. Telling a partner that they are crossing a relationship boundary can be a difficult thing to do, so developing effective communication skills is a really important part of relationships education.

Ask the young people to think of a boundary or limitation which is important to them. Using the worksheet, they can write this down as a scenario. Next ask them to think about how they would approach this conversation respectfully while ensuring they are being listened to.

Communicating my boundaries

Practice scenario:
What to say/what to do:
Practice scenario:
What to say/what to do:

UNHEALTHY RELATIONSHIPS

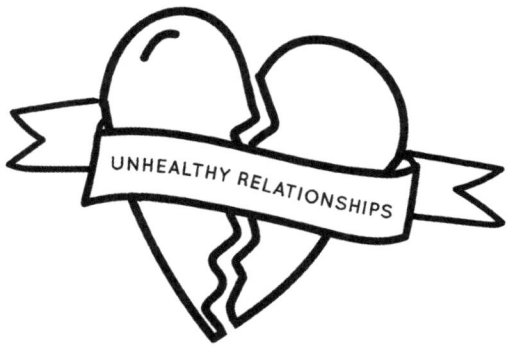

Introducing the topic: Teaching young people to recognize the warning signs of an unhealthy relationship can help to prevent teen relationship abuse. Many of the unhealthy relationship traits and behaviours we see among young people are often confused with signs of love, for example signs of extreme jealousy and possessiveness. The following activity can help young people identify unhealthy relationship traits.

When delivering this topic with groups, I have used excerpts from the young adult novel *The Places I've Cried in Public*, by Holly Bourne, as this provides a great introduction to new and emerging words such as gaslighting. Poetry or quotes from R.M. Drake and Lauren Bowman can be very thought provoking and are particularly useful for exploring break-ups.

Video clips from recent and age-relevant reality TV programmes or soaps, which show unhealthy relationship behaviours such as arguments, gossiping, controlling behaviours and jealousy, can be easily sourced from YouTube. For photographs, I have used media images or campaign posters on the topic of unhealthy relationships. A quick web search or providing a physical copy of a newspaper or magazine can be great.

Relationship quotes can often be found by searching the hashtag #relationshipquotes on social media; many have been beautifully illustrated and can be printed.

ACTIVITY: SILENCE AND STICKY NOTES

Break pupils into small groups of three or more, and provide each group with a stimulus or discussion prompt. This could be a photograph, video clip, quote, or excerpt from a book. You can choose to give each group the same stimulus, particularly if you are short of time, but if possible it is good to provide a variety linked to the same topic.

This activity works best when the young people are working in smaller groups as it encourages everyone to contribute. Each group will also need a large sheet of paper for the desk.

Place the quote, iPad, photograph, book excerpts in the middle of the paper and supply lots of sticky notes and felt-tip pens. The idea is to get the group to think about the prompt for themselves, writing their individual responses on to sticky notes and placing these on the large piece of paper. It is important to encourage quiet while the group do this, as it can help to engage young people who wouldn't ordinarily join in a group discussion, and also adds to the emotiveness and seriousness of the topic.

Allow time for all of the young people to consider their thoughts and contribute something, before encouraging them to read the statements from others in their group and write a written response to all of the comments. The idea is to encourage young people to have an open and honest conversation, ask questions and provoke thought, and, if they would like to respectfully agree or disagree, to do this silently. The groups can then walk around and look at other groups' prompts and comments. This is similar to a gallery walk, but at this stage the young people are not asked to add anything, but to think of a question they could ask another group. The final part of the activity is the question-and-answer aspect where the groups talk about their prompt and the thinking this brought about for them.

TEEN RELATIONSHIP ABUSE

Introducing the topic: Abuse in teenage relationships is when a young person begins to feel scared or controlled by the person they're with. Abuse in relationships can happen to anyone, regardless of age, gender or family situations. It can happen to boys and girls and to teenagers in same-sex relationships.

WOULD YOU SPOT THE SIGNS OF AN ABUSIVE RELATIONSHIP?

RELATIONSHIPS

HEALTHY SIGNS

OPEN COMMUNICATION
QUALITY TIME TOGETHER
SHARED VALUES
MUTUAL RESPECT
REALISTIC EXPECTATIONS
ONGOING SUPPORT
STRONG SENSE OF TRUST
MAKING SHARED DECISIONS
YOU FEEL SAFE
YOU ACCEPT EACH OTHER
YOU HAVE FUN
HEALTHY BOUNDARIES
MUTUAL AFFECTION
YOU ENJOY TIME APART
HEALTHY DISAGREEMENTS
YOU FEEL A SENSE OF BELONGING
YOU INSPIRE EACH OTHER TO BE BETTER

WARNING SIGNS

GUILT TRIPS
WITHDRAWAL OF AFFECTION
ISOLATES YOU FROM FAMILY
USING MONEY TO CONTROL
UNREASONABLE JEALOUSY
IGNORING OR EXCLUDING YOU
REFUSES TO COMMUNICATE
GASLIGHTING OR MANIPULATION
CONSTANT PUT-DOWNS
HUMILIATES OR EMBARASSES YOU
SAYING "I LOVE YOU... BUT"
USES THREATS OR IMTIMIDATION
BLAMES YOU
COMPULSIVE LYING
NAME CALLING
USES FORCE TO CONTROL YOU
REGULARLY CRITICISES YOU
THREATENS VIOLENCE OR SUICIDE

@ TOUGHCOOKIESED

A 2018 report carried out by Women's Aid and *Cosmopolitan* magazine highlighted that a third of teenage girls have been in an abusive relationship.

The research also found that when the other two-thirds of girls who said they had not experienced relationship abuse were asked further questions, the results increased to 64 per cent of the girls having experienced abusive behaviour – they just didn't realize it.

Another report, *Young People's Attitudes to Violence Against Women: Report on Findings from the Young People in Scotland Survey 2014* (Local Government and Communities Direc-torate 2016), explored young people's attitudes towards domestic violence and abuse and found that while the majority of young people view violence and abuse negatively, some young people suggested that depending on the situation, they would consider some types of abuse to be acceptable.

ACTIVITY: MEGAN'S STORY

Give a copy of Megan's story to the young people, one person or you could read it aloud. Allow some time for reflection before beginning the questioning and discussion.

MEGAN'S STORY

I wasn't really sure what I had done wrong. One minute I was laughing along with friends, mutual friends, and then next, I knew, I just knew. I could feel the energy. When we walked off, he mentioned it straight away. 'What was all that about?' he said, 'You think I can't see what you are doing?'

I used to like his jealousy; it made me feel special for a while. Like, it was a way that I could know and feel as if he really loved me. But then it just got really awkward and would make me feel worried and anxious about just being myself.

Was I being overly friendly with our friends? I wondered, even though I knew deep down I wasn't. Tired of feeling as if I couldn't even be myself anymore, I turned and said to him, 'You're paranoid, it's not my fault, I did nothing wrong.' He grabbed me by the hair, put his head to my face and shouted with gritted teeth, 'What, what?' He grabbed my phone and threw it on the floor and then just stormed off.

I picked up my phone, the screen was cracked again. I would have to make another excuse about why and my parents would be in a mood with me about me not being responsible and not looking after my things.

I hated this. I ran after him, holding in my tears, as he would just be more annoyed if I cried. I knew he would calm down eventually and we would be okay and he would say sorry, and then things would be really, really good again. That's what he did last time.

Ask the young people to either share aloud or write down their initial thoughts about Megan's story. What do they think about the way Megan has dealt with the situation? What do they think about the behaviour of Megan's partner? Do they think that this is relationship abuse?

ACTIVITY: SPOTTING SIGNS OF AN ABUSIVE RELATIONSHIP

With the young people working as a whole group task them to list some of the things they would perceive to be violent or abusive. Encourage them to think more broadly to also include emotional forms of abuse which are sometimes overlooked by teens.

Explore the reasons why some young people may view violence or abuse as acceptable: talk about cheating and the act of self-defence, which are often two of the most common answers from my discussions with young people. Does being cheated on warrant violence? What would be a safer way to respond? How can young people better deal with their feelings when angry, let down and hurt? Why do some young people not recognize emotional abuse behaviour as a type of abuse?

The Teen Power and Control Wheel, developed by the Domestic Abuse Intervention Project in Duluth, Minnesota, is a useful tool, freely available to download, which can help young people understand further aspects of relationships abuse. The inside parts of the wheel diagram describe the subtle, continual behaviours which can happen over time, while the outer circle represents physical and sexual violence.

Role play

Before using role play, it is helpful to establish or revisit your ground rules for RSE.

Download and print the role-play cards and cut them out, ensuring that there are enough for one scenario card per group. Provide pen and paper for notes and planning.

Break the young people into groups and allow them time to familiarize themselves with their given role-play card. Encourage them to think about what characters their role play will need, in order for them to develop a scene and showcase the type of relationship abuse they have been given. Provoke them to also think about the bystanders and other people who may be witness to it. Ensure that everyone in the group has a role.

Remind the groups that the task is to act out a scenario, and for the other groups to try to spot any signs of relationship abuse or violence.

Tell the young people to develop each of their characters, thinking about how they might feel and react, how they would speak, what their body language would look like, where they might be, who may witness the abuse and who could help them.

Allow time for the young people to rehearse the role plays before performing them to others.

Following each role play, ask the groups to say which type of abuse they spotted. Discuss in more depth how the characters reacted, how they felt and what they did as a result. If you have time you could end with hot seating; where the young people stay in character and are questioned by the group. Do this individually or in groups.

Encourage some of the groups to conclude the role plays with positive solutions and outcomes.

⊻ Role-play cards

Emotional abuse: controlling behaviour, such as telling someone where they can go and what they can wear. Isolating them so they are no longer spending time with their circle of friends or family.

Online abuse: threatening to post personal pictures or information about them.

Controlling someone's finances: withholding money or stopping someone going to work.

Snooping: reading emails, text messages or letters.

Sexual abuse: making someone do something sexual when they don't want to. (You don't need to act out the sexual activity – think of more appropriate ways you could show this is happening, maybe using words, conversations, setting the scene.)

Physical abuse: violence towards someone, such as kicking, punching, hitting. (You don't need to act out the violent activity – think of more appropriate ways you could show this is happening, maybe using noise, choreographing a fake punch.)

ACTIVITY: GETTING HELP AND HELPING OTHERS

Ask the groups to think about what they would do if they were worried that a friend was in an abusive relationship or living in a family where one adult was being abusive to another?

Explain about local and national helplines they could call and who they could speak to at school or in the community.

Encourage the class to list five people or places young people could go to get help.

◆ Chapter 7 ◆

Sex Education

INTRODUCTION

In this section, you will find a range of age-appropriate and relevant activities which will help you to deliver an engaging programme of sex education covering a range of topics, including the human body, safeguarding and sexual health.

In the 2013 Ofsted Report, *Not Yet Good Enough*, young people described their sex education as 'too little, too late and too biological', so it is important that when developing a programme for sex education that the needs of young people are met and they receive information about their growing and changing bodies and health awareness before they face these situations in real life.

According to a study which looks closely at the changing sexual attitudes and behaviour of the British population (Lewis *et al.* 2017), most heterosexual young people have sexual intercourse for the first time at the age of 16, and research indicates that this has not changed much over the last few decades. Much less is known about when young people start having sexual activities of any kind, including kissing.

The study also suggests that more young people are engaging in different types of sex, such as oral and anal sex. It is important, therefore, that the sex education lessons we provide include reference to this and do not only focus on the teachings of penis in vagina sex.

Language will also be an important aspect of sex education, so consider what you will say and do to ensure you do not assume gender or sexuality, or reinforce sexist stereotypes. Familiarize yourself beforehand with key information about the naming of body parts, contraceptive options and any relevant legislation. It can be helpful to have a one-page fact sheet on hand, and so we have included a number of these in this section.

CONDOM DEMO

Putting a condom on a banana is what most people assume sex educators do for a living, but you will not find that activity in this book. When carrying out and demonstrating safe condom use, I would suggest purchasing a condom demonstrator rather than using fruit. Of course, sex education should be funny and I encourage you to use humour often as part of your delivery, and absolutely make time for and allow young people to laugh – but also remember that the sessions, workshops and activities you provide are likely to be the only face-to-face sex education most young people will get. Finding the right balance of entertainment and education is key.

Think carefully about how you might deal with any silliness which may arise and revisit your ground rules again and again. Where possible, try not to remove a young person from the group. Ask yourself, if they do miss out on these learning opportunities, how likely are they to get the chance to participate in learning about the topic again?

Fertility education, including the menopause, is a topic which now features in the new Relationship and Sex Education and Health Education guidance. The need for this was backed up by a number of health and education professionals, who were becoming increasingly concerned with the lack of knowledge people had about the age-related decline in fertility.

A national survey of 1000 16–24-year-olds (male and female) commissioned specifically for the Fertility Education Initiative Task Force (2016) found worrying gaps in knowledge about fertility and reproductive health.

Good and effective fertility education includes:

- learning about human reproduction, the male and female reproductive system from puberty to menopause
- understanding what fertility and infertility mean and knowing the signs, symptoms and preventable causes of fertility issues, such as the impact of untreated sexually transmitted infections, drug use and obesity.

In order to remain inclusive, fertility education should also understand modern families and be aware of the many options available to become parents, such as assisted conception techniques, used by both heterosexual, LGBTQIA + and single people. Other routes to parenthood (such as adoption, fostering, step families) and having the choice to live life without children should also be mentioned.

SEXUALLY TRANSMITTED INFECTIONS

It can be difficult to make the teaching of sexually transmitted infections fun and engaging, and over the years I have tried and tested many approaches to this. In the beginning of my career as a sex educator, scare tactics were often used, sharing images of worst-case scenario STIs with the intention to put young people off taking risks. But more recently, debate among educators and evaluation from young people have shown mixed feelings towards this approach. Although many young people enjoy the gruesomeness of being shown images of the advanced stages of sexually transmitted diseases, there are questions about the value of this. The main factor is whether this exposure is changing behaviour. Through my own evaluation, I would say it is not, and that it is more likely to give young people who may be at risk of an STI an air of confidence that they are okay.

What has worked well in my teaching about sexually transmitted infections has been to ensure that the lessons also include information about testing, not just symptoms.

Young people are often put off by the idea that tests can be painful and invasive and so addressing any misunderstandings they have about this can be helpful. If possible, it can be good to link up with genitourinary medicine (GUM) or chlamydia screening services, which can support young people to feel more confident in accessing these places, should they need to.

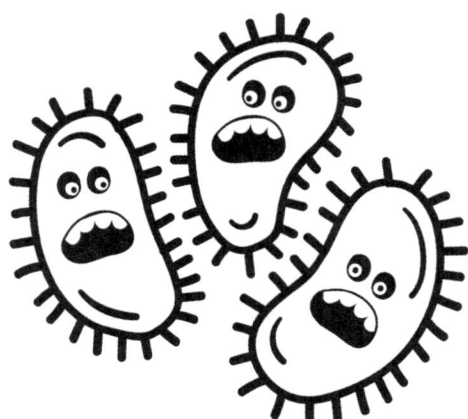

Teaching about pleasure should also be embedded in the delivery of sex education. I think sometimes when people hear me say that, the assumption is I am asking them to teach about how to make sex good, in a magazine 'try this position of the month' type of way. But it's not. Teaching teens about pleasure is an important aspect of consent, power and equality. It is about empowering young people, developing positive self-esteem, building confidence and their understanding their own right to body autonomy, enabling them to know what their relationship and sexual activity boundaries and preferences are and being able to communicate them. It also links to the mammoth task we face as sex educators to unlearn all the things young people have acquired about sex from their peers, the media and porn, which very often suggest that women orgasm, all of the time, very loudly, and through penis in vagina sex.

Sex education works best when it is proactive and when it supports the development of young people's knowledge. It should create learning opportunities where young people can practise and advance new skills, and it should provide a safe space to think about and reflect on their thoughts, beliefs and ideas as well as feelings and emotions in relation to sex.

Activities and ideas to help you teach about sex, including consent, harassment, confidentiality, fertility, different types of sex, pleasure, safe sex, contraception and pregnancy choices make up this next chapter.

THE A-Z OF SEX ED

The A–Z is a great icebreaker for sex education. This fun game is a great way to get everyone comfortable with the topic, build confidence to ask questions and increase participation. It can also be a good baseline and needs assessment tool, as the young people's answers provide an indication as to what they know, what they have heard about, what is relevant and what gaps they may have in their knowledge and understanding. I also use this to explore relationship and sex education language and terminology.

Before playing it would be a good idea to revisit ground rules. Next explain the concept of red, amber and green words. Red words are not okay to share or write down as part of the game, these words would represent words which would go against the inclusion policy and Equalities Act. Green words are words that include the correct terminology used in science and medical language. Amber words would represent slang terms, these can be offensive or inappropriate in some settings and to some members of the group. Once red, amber and green are explained, this can be used to challenge any offensive language used without the young person feeling like they are unable to explore and learn.

To play as a whole group, write the alphabet on the board and ask the group to shout out a word that they associate with sex education for each letter of the alphabet. Remember that as well as proving a fun starter, the activity also provides a safe space to explore language around sex, bodies and relationships which may be sexist, homophobic or racist. When a word is suggested that may be knowingly or unknowingly offensive, tell the young people which category from red, green or amber this fits and if possible, explain the reasons why the word cannot be used. For example, a young person may share a derogatory term which is homophobic; we would explain that this term is a homophobic slur and not one which we can include. This should not be seen as a telling off, as we are trying to create a safe learning space where dated and inappropriate language can be challenged and new more inclusive language can be learned.

Work your way through the alphabet going from A through to Z, spending time to explore some of the language and words suggested. For example, if slang terms are used, this can be a great opportunity to share the correct term. Where medical terms or inclusive language is used, this provides a great opportunity to display positive feedback which reinforces the use of these terms.

CONSENT

Introducing the topic: What is an MP and what does an MP do?

MP stands for Member of Parliament. An MP is elected to represent their constituency and speak for the people in Parliament.

In their constituency, MPs will get involved with things happening in the community. They also hold MP surgeries where local people can come along to and talk to them, ask questions and raise issues they would like discussing in Parliament.

In Parliament, the MP will voice the concerns and ask questions on behalf of their communities. MPs also attend the House of Commons to debate national issues and to vote on changes to new guidance and legislation.

In 2019, MPs voted in favour of making Relationships and Sex Education a compulsory subject in all schools in England from September 2020; 538 MPs voted for this and 21 against.

ACTIVITY: MP FOR A DAY

Ask the young people if they were an MP representing their local constituency, how would they have voted?

Have the young people practise, with all those in favour of compulsory RSE shouting 'aye' and all those against saying 'no'.

Continuing with the idea that that the young people are now Members of Parliament, task them to look more closely at the laws relating to sexual consent, including the age of consent in the UK.

Ask the young people to put themselves in the role of an MP where they would need to consider the thoughts and ideas of their constituents rather than their own personal values and to be prepared to make a vote at the end.

Break the young people into small groups giving each group a printout of the age of consent card to encourage them to explore the topic in more depth.

 ## THE AGE OF CONSENT

In the UK, the age of consent is 16. 'Consent' means to say yes. So, the 'age of consent' is when the law says a young person can make their own decision to say 'yes' or 'no' to any sexual activity. Through a show of hands, ask the young people to state if the age of consent (currently set at 16) is something they agree or disagree with and tally the answers on the board. To support the young people's understanding of the sexual activity consent law facilitate a whole group discussion and allow time for the young people to consider these questions:

- Why do you think the age of consent for sexual activity is set at 16?

Often young people will answer that they think the age of consent is set at 16 due to puberty and the maturity of young people, but they should also consider teenage parenthood and the impact on education. Explain to young people how the age of consent law has been developed to protect children. Also use this opportunity to explain clearly how any sexual contact without consent is illegal, regardless of the age of those involved and that children under the age of 13 cannot give consent to any type of sexual activity.

- In other countries across the world the age of consent is lower and in others it is higher, and some countries don't have an age of consent law at all; what do you think are the positives and negatives of this?
- What other things relevant to young people, can you think of that have age-related laws? For example, age restrictions on gaming, smoking, purchase of alcohol, driving, getting married, tattoos and piercings, employment or joining the military and sexting (do the young people know what the sexting law is?). Compare the age of sexual consent law in relation to these other laws. What are your thoughts, would they change them?

After the discussion, go back and ask again 'do we agree or disagree with the age of consent being 16?' Have the numbers on the tally changed in any way, and if so, why?

WHAT IS SEXUAL ACTIVITY?

Introducing the topic: Consent in relationships is about each person being in control and saying yes to doing things because they would like to and not because they are feeling pressured to or are being coerced. Each person has the right to say no or change their mind if they no longer wish to continue with a sexual activity.

Many young people wrongly believe the consent law is only relevant when it comes to sexual intercourse or penetrative sex. But the law itself relates to 'sexual activity', which can include a whole spectrum of things, such as snogging, a boob grope or any kind of intimate touch.

Sexual Offences Act 2003 definition of 'sexual':

The definition of sexual is contained within section 78 of the Sexual Offences Act 2003 and applies to all offences in part 1 of the Act, with the exception of section 71 (sexual activity in a public lavatory). Penetration, touching or any other activity is sexual if a reasonable person would consider that: whatever its circumstances or any person's purpose in relation to it, it is because of its nature sexual, or because of its nature it may be sexual and because of its circumstances or the purpose of any person in relation to it (or both) it is sexual. (Rape and Sexual Offences 2021)

ACTIVITY: SEXUAL ACTIVITY SPECTRUM

The activity is designed to support young people to understand that consent is a necessity for all kinds of sexual activity.

Ask each young person to take a sticky note and on this write down something which they think could be deemed a sexual activity. Once they have written down their idea they should take it to the spectrum of consent and place the sticky note where they think it may go. The spectrum of consent should be a visible line, which starts at one side with 'No consent is required' and finishes on the other side with 'You must have consent'. The activity works well when you use a line of string, pegs and card.

Suggestions for differentiation: Sometimes groups of young people can feel uncomfortable putting forward their ideas for sexual activity; if you feel this could be the case for your groups you could create the sexual activity cards yourself in advance and have the young people sort them out.

TALKING POINTS

Consent is about communication. It needs to happen every time for every type of sexual activity. Giving consent to one type of sexual activity does not mean you have given consent for other types of sexual activity. An example of this is if a person agrees to kiss someone (consent), that doesn't mean that the other person has permission to take off their clothes while kissing them.

With sexual consent, it is important to discuss boundaries and expectations. When would be the best time to discuss this?

COMMUNICATING CONSENT

Introducing: the topic: Let's begin by talking about 'No means No', which is most definitely an important aspect of consent, but not really just what consent is about. Before any sexual activity takes place, the focus of consent should be on whether the person has communicated their boundaries and said yes.

ACTIVITY: QUICK-FIRE QUESTIONS

- Why is consent not about making your move and waiting for a person to say no? (If this was to happen a person could be touched without their consent.)
- Who is responsible for consent? (The person who is making the move.)

Within sex education, consent is considered to be about communication that is clear, freely given, enthusiastic, mutual, ongoing and something that you get and give before any sexual activity takes place.

Clear: Has the person said 'yes' to the sexual activity they have been asked to do? Consent should not be assumed. The person should make it clear they are happy to continue, and consent shouldn't feel unsure. There are usually lots of non-verbal cues which show if a person is interested or maybe uncomfortable, but body language alone should not be relied on as clear consent.

Freely given: For consent to be freely given, neither person should feel coerced, pressured, threatened or bullied.

Enthusiastic: Enthusiastic participation in sexual activity is a must.

Mutual: Both partners need to agree with what is happening and going to happen; communicating boundaries and listening to each other is an important part of consent.

Ongoing: Consent is an ongoing thing; before you do something else it is important to keep checking in and making sure that you have an enthusiastic yes for that too.

ACTIVITY: CONSENT AND PIZZA

Introduce the concept that sex is, in some ways, quite like pizza! Pizza, like sex, comes in lots of different shapes and sizes. There are so many varieties, which means that when you think about pizza there is no guarantee that the kind of pizza you are thinking of — the base, the sauce, the toppings, the crust – is going to be identical to that in the thoughts of the person sitting next to you. And that's the same when it comes to sex.

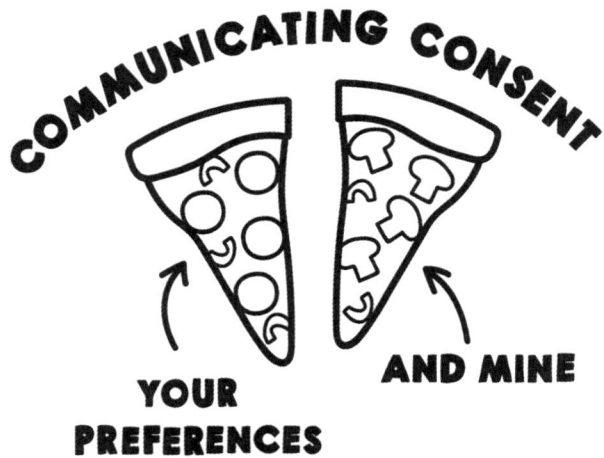

Ask the young people to take a piece of card and a pen (they should not show what they are writing to anyone else) and jot down their idea of the perfect pizza. Encourage them to be super descriptive, thinking about the choices they have for a base: stone baked, deep pan, thin and crispy. Do they need a gluten-free base? Will their pizza have stuffed crust? Will it be stuffed with cheese, or tomato or something else? What size will their pizza be? Will it be 15cm, 25cm or more? Will their pizza be a fresh pizza, made from scratch? Or are they thinking of a favourite pizza brand, ready-made, for the oven, in the microwave or toaster? Maybe they are thinking of a takeaway pizza, ordered from their favourite restaurant. What about the toppings: will these be tomato or BBQ sauce, cheese, ham, pineapple, pepperoni, chicken, peppers, mushroom, onion, sweetcorn? Would they like oil on it, garlic infused or something else? Or maybe they don't even like pizza! They might have written down something else. Encourage the young people to think about whether there is one which they absolutely do not like and would never eat. Get them to make a note of this too.

Ask them to pop their card safely to one side – they will come back to it.

Explain to the young people that communicating our preferences, boundaries, likes and dislikes is an important part of consent. But some of them may feel awkward about this. The reason for this could be down to where they have learned and what they understand about sex.

Ask the young people where they learned about sex – what it looks like, who initiates, how it happens, and what you do. Most young people will answer that they learned most of what they know from the media. And most media sex scenes don't show sexual consent. Ask the young people if they can think of a time when they have seen consent clearly communicated in the media.

Share a clip of kissing scenes taken from the media. One video which works well is Disney's *Top Ten Kisses*, which can be found on YouTube. Ask the young people to watch and to make notes of where clear and enthusiastic consent is being communicated. You will often find that there isn't any. Young people will often suggest here that consent has been given and that it was shown or given through non-verbal communication.

Revisit the notes on what consent is and should be: consent is considered to be about communication that is clear, freely given, enthusiastic, mutual, ongoing and something that you get and give before any sexual activity takes place.

For the next part of the activity, the young people are going to practise their consent communication skills.

They will now need the detailed and descriptive notes they made earlier about their pizza choices; these are going to be used as an example of their preferences and their boundaries.

Ask the young people to work in pairs and communicate their pizza preferences and boundaries to each other using non-verbal communication. The non-verbal communication can include only facial expressions and hand gestures.

Reflect with the young people on this activity: how easy or difficult was it to clearly communicate their choices and preferences using non-verbal communication?

Try the activity once again, this time asking the young people to use verbal communication.

Reflect on the differences; was it easier to verbally say what they liked and disliked? Was it easier to know they had been understood? Were they able to voice their no-go areas?

ACTIVITY: HOW TO TALK ABOUT CONSENT

Task the young people to write down their examples of the language they could use to have an open and honest talk about consent. For example, they could say things like:

- I'd really like to…
- Are you okay with that?
- Does this feel good?
- I really like you but I'm not ready for that right now.

SEXUAL HARASSMENT

Introducing the topic: Sexual harassment is a type of bullying intended to hurt or intimidate someone. It includes verbal sexual harassment, such as making sexual jokes about a person or saying and writing sexual comments, as well as physical sexual harassment, such as making sexual gestures, touching a person in a sexual way without their consent. Sexual harassment can happen in person, via text or online and includes asking someone to share sexual pictures, sending someone unwanted sexual pictures or starting sexual rumours about a person.

ACTIVITY: SEXUAL HARASSMENT OR FLIRTY BANTER?

 Download and print the cards and distribute them among the young people. Ask them to read the cards and decide if these situations would be flirtatious banter or sexual harassment.

Being repeatedly asked to go on a date. You have made it clear you are not interested and have said no many times.
Every time you walk into form, another student makes orgasm noises. This makes you feel really embarrassed.
While walking up the stairs, someone grabs hold of your bra strap and pulls it.
You are working a weekend job, and you are the only male. While packing up at the end of your shift you overhear a group of female workers telling sexual jokes and sharing stories about sex – they are not saying it to you, but it is making you feel uncomfortable.
You are trying to make your way home from a dance class, and are at the changing room door ready to leave but the young, attractive dance teacher, who you do actually really like and are attracted to, is purposely standing in the doorway and blocking your exit.

A student in the year above you at school has sent you messages via social media, which are of a sexual nature.
That's what she said.
When walking home from the youth club you pass a shop and on a few occasions the people who work there have made sexualized comments about your body and what you are wearing.
You are at a music festival and someone in the crowd behind you takes a photograph up your skirt.

TALKING POINTS

All of the statements on the cards could be sexual harassment. How do the young people feel about that?

It can be easy to dismiss sexual harassment as just flirtatious banter, especially if we think about the person doing these types of behaviours being someone we quite like and are attracted to.

If someone you like and are attracted to places their hand on your knee, sends you a flirty text or announces they like you in that way too, it can make you feel great if that behaviour is wanted. But when these situations happen from the wrong person or at the wrong time, the situation can become creepy, uncomfortable and even make you feel ashamed.

ACTIVITY: JARGON BUSTER

The Concise Oxford Dictionary of Current English defines sexual harassment as any 'unwanted sexual advances, obscene remarks, etc.' (Fowler 2012).

And the Equality Act 2010 says it's an 'unwanted conduct of a sexual nature' which violates a person's dignity or 'creates an intimidating, hostile, degrading or offensive environment' (Equality Act 2010).

A government report (Department for Education 2021) looking at sexual harassment in schools describes it as 'unwanted conduct of a sexual nature' that can occur online and offline. It states:

Sexual harassment can include:

- sexual comments, such as: telling sexual stories, making lewd comments, making sexual remarks about clothes and appearance and calling someone sexualised names;
- sexual 'jokes' or taunting;
- physical behaviour, such as: deliberately brushing against someone, interfering with someone's clothes (schools and colleges should be considering when any of this crosses a line into sexual violence – it is important to talk to and consider the experience of the victim) and displaying pictures, photos or drawings of a sexual nature; and
- online sexual harassment. This may be standalone, or part of a wider pattern of sexual harassment and/or sexual violence. It may include:
  - non-consensual sharing of sexual images and videos;
  - sexualised online bullying;
  - unwanted sexual comments and messages, including on social media; and
  - sexual exploitation; coercion and threats.

Task the pupils to write a jargon-free paragraph which explains what sexual harassment is, in a way that could make it easier and better understood by young people.

UPSKIRTING

Introducing the topic: One of the kinds of sexual harassment situations from the cards describes the offence of upskirting.

The Upskirting Act, which is more commonly known as the Voyeurism (Offences) Act, came into force on 12 April 2019.

'Upskirting' is where someone takes a picture under a person's clothing (not necessarily a skirt) without their permission and or knowledge, with the intention of viewing their genitals or buttocks (with or without underwear) to obtain sexual gratification or cause the victim humiliation, distress or alarm. It is a criminal offence. And a person, of any gender, can be a victim.

The act was introduced following an 18-month campaign by activist Gina Martin, who herself was a victim of upskirting.

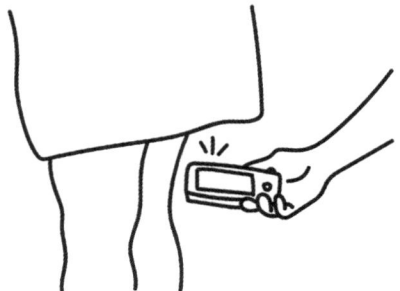

With the young people, research Gina's story and campaign. (A great article documenting Gina's experience can be found on the *Teen Vogue* website titled 'How my traumatic experience with upskirting taught me how to be an activist' (Nast 2021). There is also a TED talk which would be useful to watch, called 'They told me to change my clothes. I changed the law instead' (Martin 2020).)

You could include other campaigns aiming to end sexual harassment, such as the MeToo movement.

You could also share information about the UK government's commitment to preventing and ending peer-on-peer sexual harassment in schools.

ACTIVITY: SOCIAL ACTION CAMPAIGNS

Social action is about making change, and there are lots of ways this can happen. It can include individual action, such as reflecting on our own values and behaviours, developing better skills and becoming more informed. It can include group work, where people come together with others and raise awareness through events and campaigns, and it can include communities, where larger groups of people may work together to bring about change, for example through peaceful protest or speaking to Parliament.

Task the group to create a campaign that will educate other young people about sexual harassment in schools. They could create posters, badges and t-shirts, or they could interview people for a podcast or a video.

They just need to get creative and make a change.

CONFIDENTIALITY

Introducing the topic: Confidentiality involves a situation in which you expect someone to keep information secret. The following statements may be seen:

- They signed a confidentiality agreement.
- All letters will be treated with complete confidentiality.
- He was fired for a breach of confidentiality (a situation where secret information was told to someone else).

Did you know that young people are entitled to the same confidentiality as adults? This means that health professionals and other workers providing relationships and sexual health information, advice or guidance to young people have a duty to not disclose anything a young person has discussed with them without the young person's consent.

Why might this be an important factor for young people and young people's health services?

Confidentiality can be very important to young people, particularly to those teens who may be anxious about seeking sexual health advice, fearing what they discuss won't be kept private and parents and carers could be informed.

However, confidentiality policies that are held in most young people's services mean that even if a young person is under 16, their information will still be kept in confidence and not shared with anyone else. The only exception to this is if the worker they speak to feels that the young person could be in harm or danger. This is referred to as safeguarding or child protection, which means that young people under 16 are entitled to special protection from harm. If a worker speaks to a young person and is worried about them, and needs to pass on and share this information with someone else, they should in most circumstances discuss this with the young person first.

GILLICK COMPETENCY AND FRASER GUIDELINES

The Gillick competency and Fraser guidelines help people who work with children to balance the need to listen to children's wishes with the responsibility to keep them safe.

FRASER GUIDELINES

Fraser guidelines provide direction on giving advice and treatment to young people under 16 years of age. These state that sexual health services can be offered without parental consent providing that:

→ the young person understands the advice that is being given

→ the young person cannot be persuaded to inform or seek support from their parents, and will not allow the worker to inform the parents that contraceptive/protection, for example condom advice, is being given

→ the young person is likely to begin or continue to have sexual intercourse without contraception or protection by a barrier method

→ the young person's physical or mental health is likely to suffer unless they receive contraceptive advice or treatment

→ it is in the young person's best interest to receive contraceptive/safe sex advice and treatment without parental consent.

GILLICK COMPETENCY

Gillick competency applies to young people receiving medical advice but it is also used by educators in other settings. There is no set of defined questions to assess Gillick competency. Professionals need to consider several things when assessing a child's capacity to consent, including:

→ the child's age, maturity and mental capacity

→ their understanding of the issue and what it involves – including advantages, disadvantages and potential long-term impact

→ their understanding of the risks, implications and consequences that may arise from their decision

→ how well they understand any advice or information they have been given

→ their understanding of any alternative options, if available

→ their ability to explain a rationale around their reasoning and decision-making.

GETTING SUPPORT AND HELPING OTHERS

ACTIVITY: USEFUL PEOPLE AND PLACES LIST

Ask the young people to think about who they could go to for help, at home and at school. Work together to create a flipchart list of all the people and places young people can go to for help. One place that many people go to when they have questions about relationships or need help may be online. Explain that there are many places which can offer safe spaces and support (Childline, the Child Exploitation and Online Protection Centre) and some which are not that great (strangers, articles which may be sharing wrong or harmful information).

Often friends are the first people that someone will go to with a worry or concern about their relationships or sex. This is largely due to the fact that they trust them enough to talk about their experience, and know that the friend will be there to help and get support. Some young people who want information, advice or guidance about their relationship or sexual health might need help from a friend when talking to a trusted adult.

ACTIVITY: PASS IT ON

Explain to the young people that you are going to think about how serious or small a problem is because that will help them to think about what they can do to solve it, and whether to seek help from others or not. Start by asking each member of the group to write down on a sticky note a common issue or problem relating to growing up, relationships or sex and health that young people may face. This may include situations like breaking up with a partner, worrying about a missed period, finding out they are pregnant, not starting puberty when other friends have, a controlling partner, worries about the way their body looks, STI symptoms, feeling pressured to do something in a relationship, or sharing nudes with a partner and regretting it. On the board draw a table with four squares:

Deal with it	How?
Pass it on	Who to?

Using the young people's situations, ask them to come up individually and place their sticky note where they think it should go on the table, explaining that it is sometimes very important to seek adult help. Times when this should happen include when someone is sick or hurt or when something unsafe is happening. It is also important to get adult help if something is happening to make a person feel bullied or scared, especially if this problem lasts for a long time. A good indicator of when to ask for help is when a person feels the problem is too big to solve on their own, and they may need specialist help, like from a doctor, the police or a social worker. They should use this advice to help make their decision.

If the young person feels the situation is something that they feel they have the skills and knowledge to deal with, ask them how they might help. Ask them to also suggest a response. They may say things such as listening, offering their own advice, being a shoulder to cry on, or seeking and finding more information, for example visiting a young person-friendly website for more advice. If the young person feels the situation requires them to pass it on, then ask them to think about who they would pass it on to and why.

Once completed and everyone has had their turn, speak to the group about confidentiality and what it means to break the confidentiality of a friend. Many young people feel concerned about letting down their friends and so instead of speaking up and getting their friends help when it is needed, they worry about what might happen to their friendship. Explain to the young people about the concept of safeguarding and when it is okay to break confidentiality. Help the young people understand why it is sometimes necessary and how this can be very important in keeping each other safe.

SAFE SEX

Introducing the topic: Alongside consent, safe sex also includes making sure young people are protected from sexually transmitted infections, and that they are taking care of their own and their partner's sexual health. This includes learning about contraception, and preventing unplanned pregnancies.

Figures released by Public Health England for 2018–2019 (Mitchell *et al.* 2020) show that there were 468,342 new STI diagnoses made at sexual health services. Young people aged under 25 continue to be the group most affected by STIs.

The most commonly diagnosed STIs in 2019 were:

- chlamydia (229,411; 49 per cent of all diagnoses)
- gonorrhoea (70,936; 15 per cent of all diagnoses)
- genital warts (51,274; 11 per cent of all diagnoses)
- genital herpes (34,570; 7 per cent of all diagnoses).

HIV stands for human immunodeficiency virus. It is a virus which attacks the immune system, which is the body's system that stops us from getting ill. If HIV is left untreated it can lead to the body becoming unable to fight off infections, and when this happens and a person becomes unwell with an infection they cannot fight off, it is called late stage HIV or AIDS. While there is no cure for HIV, a person living with HIV and taking anti-viral medication can continue to live a happy life and will not develop AIDS.

Test your young people's knowledge about the most common STIs by getting them to fill in the blanks in the STI quiz.

ACTIVITY: FILL-IN-THE-BLANKS STI QUIZ

1. Most people with this STI do not notice any symptoms and do not know they have it. It is passed on through unprotected sex (sex without a condom) and is particularly common in sexually active teenagers and young adults. . . . . is one of the most common sexually transmitted infections in the UK and it can be effectively treated with antibiotics.

2. Typical symptoms of this STI include a thick green or yellow discharge from the vagina or penis, pain when peeing and, in women, bleeding between periods. But around one in ten infected men and almost half of infected women do not experience any symptoms. . . . . is a bacterial infection.

3. A doctor or nurse can usually diagnose . . . . by looking at them. Treatments options include cream or liquid, surgery or freezing. There is no cure for this STI, but it is possible for your body to fight the virus over time. The virus can be passed

on even when there are no visible symptoms. You can get the virus from skin-to-skin contact, including vaginal and anal sex, sharing sex toys and oral sex.

4. . . . . is an STI passed on through vaginal, anal and oral sex. Treatment from a sexual health clinic can help. Symptoms can include small blisters and sores around the genitals, anus, thighs or bottom, tingling, burning or itching around the genital area, and pain when you pee. Women may also notice an unusual discharge. There is no cure for this infection but antiviral medicine and cream can be given to stop the symptoms getting worse.

5. This virus can be transmitted by vaginal, anal or oral sex, and by sharing needles, or it can be passed on from a mother to an unborn baby. To protect yourself from . . . . you should use a condom every time you have vaginal, anal or oral sex. If a person living with this virus is having treatment they can develop an undetectable viral load, and can no longer pass this on.

Answers:

1. Chlamydia	2. Gonorrhoea	3. Genital warts
4. Genital herpes	5. HIV	

CONTRACEPTION

Introducing the topic: Contraception aims to prevent pregnancy. A woman may get pregnant if a man's sperm reaches one of her eggs. Contraception tries to stop this happening by keeping the egg and sperm apart, or by stopping egg production, or by stopping a fertilized egg attaching to the lining of the womb.

Understanding contraception, how it is used and works, will involve the young people gaining good knowledge of the reproductive system, and the male and female anatomy. Before beginning sessions about contraception, it would be helpful to revisit learning about naming body parts and their functions. Activities covering this are featured in the Health Education chapter of Part 2 in this book.

Contraception is available free from the NHS in the UK, but in other countries around the world women may have to pay for contraceptive services and medications. There are 15 contraceptive methods to choose from, which include barrier methods and long-acting reversible contraceptives (LARCs). There are also permanent methods of contraception.

These are the 15 methods of contraception:

1. Caps
2. Combined pill
3. Condoms (female/internal) – barrier method
4. Condoms (male/external) – barrier method
5. Contraceptive implant – LARC
6. Contraceptive injection – LARC
7. Contraceptive patch
8. Diaphragms
9. Intrauterine device (IUD) – LARC
10. Ontrauterine system (IUS) – LARC
11. Natural family planning
12. Progestogen-only pill
13. Vaginal ring
14. Female sterilization – permanent method of contraception
15. Male sterilization, sometimes called a vasectomy – permanent method.

Other ways to prevent pregnancy could be to delay sex or have other types of sex.

Barrier methods include internal and external condoms and protect against both STIs and pregnancy.

LARCs are types of contraception which don't rely upon a person remembering to take or use it regularly for it to be effective. LARCs include the contraceptive implant IUD, IUS and the contraceptive injection.

ACTIVITY: WHAT AM I?

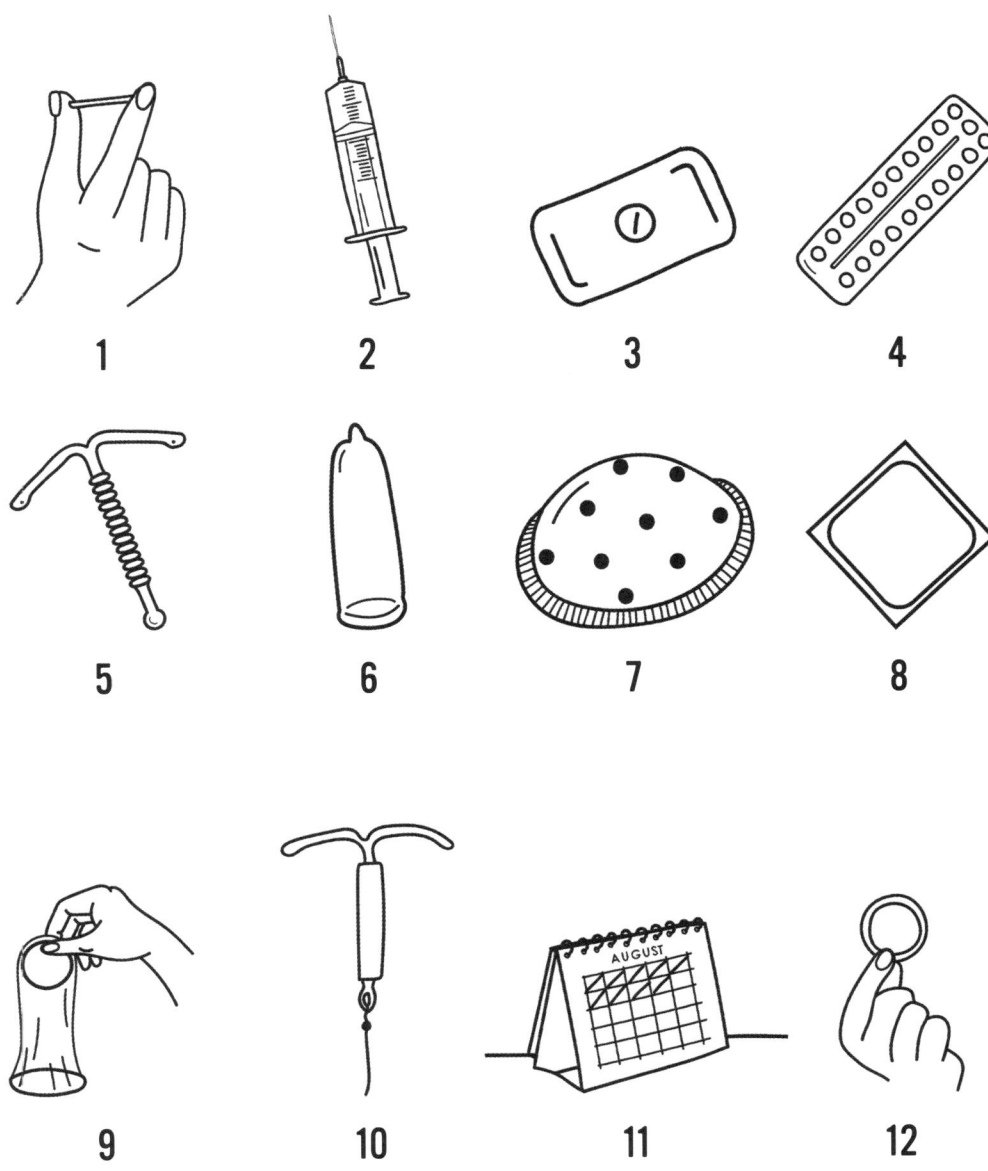

Download the illustrations of the contraceptive methods and hand the sheets out to the young people. Ask them to try and name each type of contraception. Do they know how and when it is used, how effective each method is and what the pros and cons may be?

Task the young people with making a mind map of all that they know, and check their answers.

What am I – answers

Image 1: Contraceptive implant

The contraceptive implant is a long-acting reversible contraceptive. It is a small, flexible plastic rod that is inserted under the skin in the upper arm in a procedure carried out by a doctor or nurse.

The implant releases the hormone progestogen into the bloodstream to prevent pregnancy and lasts for around three years. The implant is more than 99 per cent effective.

Advantages of the implant:

- It works for three years.
- It doesn't interrupt sex.
- It may help reduce heavy periods or period pain.

Disadvantages of the implant:

- It doesn't protect against STIs.
- There can be temporary side effects during the first few months, like headaches, nausea, breast tenderness and mood swings.
- Periods may become irregular or stop altogether.
- It requires a small procedure to have it fitted and removed.

Image 2: Contraceptive injection

The contraceptive injection releases the hormone progestogen into the bloodstream to prevent pregnancy. It lasts for 8 or 13 weeks (depending on which injection you have). It's very useful for women who find it difficult to remember to take a pill at the same time every day.

Advantages of the injection:

- Each injection lasts for either 8 or 13 weeks.
- It's an option for those who can't use oestrogen-based contraception.

Disadvantages of the injection:

- Periods can change and become irregular, heavier, shorter, lighter or stop altogether – this can carry on for some months after the injection is stopped.
- It does not protect against STIs.
- There can be a delay of up to a year before periods return to normal.

Image 3: Emergency contraceptive pill

There are two main brands of emergency contraceptive pills: Levonelle and ellaOne®. Both can be accessed free of charge from clinics, GPs and some pharmacies. You can also buy the emergency contraceptive pill.

The Levonelle pill can be taken within 72 hours (three days) of having unprotected sex, but it's most effective if taken within 12 hours of having unprotected sex. The ellaOne emergency contraceptive pill can be taken within 120 hours (five days) of having unprotected sex, but it's most effective if taken as soon as possible after having unprotected sex.

The disadvantage of the contraceptive pills is that they do not protect against sexually transmitted infections. They also do not provide ongoing contraception. Some advantages are that they are free, safe and easy to use.

Image 4: Contraceptive pills

There are two types of contraceptive pill: the combined oral contraceptive pill which is often referred to as 'the pill', and the progestogen-only pill (POP). When taken correctly, contraceptive pills are over 99 per cent effective at preventing pregnancy. The standard way to take the combined pill is to take one every day for 21 days, then a break for seven days, and during this week the person will have a bleed like a period. Traditionally, the pill is taken again after seven days. But with some types of pill, no breaks or shorter breaks may be an option. The doctor or nurse will explain the options.

With the progestogen-only pill there are 28 pills in a pack. One pill is taken every day within either three or 12 hours of the same time each day, depending on which type is prescribed. There's no break between packs of pills – when you finish a pack, the next one is started.

Advantages of the contraceptive pill:

- The progestogen-only pill is useful for those who cannot take the hormone oestrogen, which is in the combined pill, or use a contraceptive patch or vaginal ring.
- Using the pill does not interrupt sex.

Disadvantages of the contraceptive pill:

- It does not protect against STIs.
- Some medicines can make it less effective.

Image 5: Intrauterine device (IUD) copper coil

An IUD is a small T-shaped plastic and copper device that is placed into the uterus by a doctor or nurse. It works to prevent pregnancy by releasing copper and can protect against pregnancy for between five and ten years. It is sometimes referred to as the coil.
Some advantages of this method of contraception:

- When inserted correctly, they are more than 99 per cent effective.
- Once an IUD is fitted, it works straight away.
- There are no hormonal side effects.

Disadvantages of an IUD:

- It may cause periods to become heavier, longer or more painful, though this often improves after a few months.

It does not protect against STIs, and so condom use is still required.

Image 6: Condom

Condoms are the only type of contraception that can both prevent pregnancy and protect against sexually transmitted infections (STIs). Condoms are made from very thin latex (rubber), polyisoprene or polyurethane and are designed to stop semen from coming into contact with a sexual partner.

When used correctly male condoms are 98 per cent effective.

Some advantages of using condoms:

- When used correctly and every time, condoms are a reliable method of preventing pregnancy and protecting both partners from STIs, including chlamydia, gonorrhoea and HIV.
- They only need to be used when having sex.
- They come in lots of colours, fits and flavours, for different types of sexual activity.
- Condoms are very strong but may split or tear if not used properly. If this happens, it's a good idea to practise putting them on to get used to using them.

Image 7: Diaphragm

A contraceptive diaphragm or cap is a circular dome made of thin, soft silicone that's inserted into the vagina before sex.

It covers the cervix so that sperm cannot get into the womb (uterus) to fertilize an egg.

Advantages of a diaphragm or cap:

- It only needs to be used when having sex.
- It can be put in at a convenient time before having sex (extra spermicide needs to be used for those who have it in for more than three hours).
- There are usually no serious associated health risks or side effects.
- The person is in control of their contraception.

Disadvantages of a diaphragm or cap:

- It's not as effective as other types of contraception, and it depends on the person remembering to use it and using it correctly.
- It does not provide reliable protection against STIs.
- It can take time to learn how to use it.

Image 8: Contraceptive patch

The contraceptive patch is a small sticky patch that releases hormones into the body through the skin to prevent pregnancy.

When used correctly, the patch is more than 99 per cent effective at preventing pregnancy.

Advantages of the contraceptive patch:

- It's very easy to use and doesn't interrupt sex.
- Unlike the combined oral contraceptive pill, the user doesn't have to think about it every day – and only has to remember to change it once a week.

Disadvantages of the contraceptive patch:

- It may be visible, depending on where it is placed.
- It can cause skin irritation, itching and soreness.
- It doesn't protect against STIs.

Image 9: Internal/Female condom

Internal or female condoms are made from soft, thin synthetic latex or latex. They're placed inside the vagina to prevent semen getting to the womb. If used correctly, internal/female condoms are 95 per cent effective.

Advantages of female condoms:

- They protect both partners against unplanned pregnancy, STIs and HIV.
- The contraception is only used when having sex.
- There are no serious side effects.

Disadvantages of female condoms:

- Some people say that putting in the condom can interrupt sex.
- It may take some practice to get comfortable using them.

Image 10: Intrauterine system (IUS) hormone coil

An IUS is a small, T-shaped plastic device that is placed into the womb (uterus) by a doctor or nurse.

It releases the hormone progestogen to prevent pregnancy occurring and depending on which brand is used it can lasts for three to five years. When inserted correctly, it is more than 99 per cent effective.

Advantages of an IUS:

- It's one of the most effective forms of contraception available in the UK.
- Periods can become lighter, shorter and less painful – they may stop completely after the first year of use.

Disadvantages of an IUS:

- Some people may experience headaches, acne and breast tenderness after having the IUS fitted, but these usually settle with time.
- Some people experience changes in mood.
- An IUS does not protect against STIs.

Image 11: Fertility awareness

Fertility awareness, sometimes referred to as 'natural family planning' is a method of contraception where the female monitors and records fertility signals which occur during the menstrual cycle to better understand when she is ovulating and more likely to get pregnant.

Sexual intercourse is then avoided at this time to reduce the risk of pregnancy. The three fertility signals that are monitored and recorded are:

- the length of the menstrual cycle
- body temperature – daily readings are required
- changes to the cervical mucus.

If the fertility awareness steps are followed consistently and correctly, this method can be up to 99 per cent effective.

Advantages of fertility awareness:

- It does not cause any side effects.
- It can be used by anyone; it can help to be properly trained and learn the requirements and techniques.

Disadvantages of fertility awareness:

- It does not protect against STIs such as chlamydia or HIV.
- Sex has to be avoided, or contraception such as condoms used, during the time when the body might get pregnant.

Image 12: Vaginal ring

The vaginal ring is a small soft, plastic ring that is placed inside the vagina. It releases a continuous dose of the hormones oestrogen and progestogen into the bloodstream to prevent pregnancy.

If used correctly, the vaginal ring is more than 99 per cent effective.

Advantages of the vaginal ring:

- The user doesn't have to think about it every day or each time they have sex.
- It may help with premenstrual symptoms.
- Period-type bleeding usually becomes lighter, more regular and less painful.

Disadvantages of the vaginal ring:

- Some people may not feel comfortable inserting or removing it from the vagina.
- It can cause spotting and bleeding in the first few months.
- It doesn't protect against STIs.

ACTIVITIES FOR USE WITH THE CONTRACEPTIVE DISPLAY PACK

If you have a contraceptive pack, display the contraception and ask the young people to draw images of the contraceptive choices, sorting them into the correct box. You could also do this activity by downloading large images of the contraceptives and making a sorting game using hoops on the floor to represent the different categories.

Draw the contraceptive choices which protect against both unplanned pregnancy and STIs	Draw the contraceptive choices which can protect against STIs
Draw any non-hormonal contraceptives	Draw any LARCs

ACTIVITY: DESIGN A CONTRACEPTION EDUCATION BOARD GAME!

Board games can be great at getting important and factual information across. They also provide opportunities to ask questions where the game players can reflect and share their thoughts. Task the young people to work in small groups to create an educational and fun game to learn about contraception. They can use aspects from other games, changing the topic and rules to suit their concept. For the question and answers, suggest that they source information about contraception from a trusted and reliable source such as the NHS website.

When they have finished designing and making their games, have them swap the games with another group and play a different game!

Encourage the young people to write a description for their game which would be perfect to feature on an online store and to ask the groups that played their game to write a review — what did the game teach them, and what do they know now that they didn't know before?

CONDOMS

Introducing the topic: Education covering the topic of safe sex needs to include information about condoms: where to buy them, how to use them, how to make informed choices and negotiate safe sex. Before teaching find out about sexual health services local to you, which young people could be signposted to. Young people need safe opportunities to learn how to correctly use a condom. If possible, demonstrate condom use for the group and provide opportunities for young people to practice too. YouTube channels run by Brook, the NHS and Amaze.org also feature useful videos which can support your teaching.

The learning should also include young people understanding and knowing what they could do in an emergency; if a condom breaks, or if sex without a condom takes place. Alongside teaching about condom awareness, speak openly and in a non-judgemental way about the emergency contraceptive methods available.

ACTIVITY: USING CONDOMS CORRECTLY

External condoms are commonly made from latex, although non-latex versions are available for people with a latex allergy. Young people aged 25 and under can get access to condoms from sexual health services. They can also be purchased from shops and chemists. The condom acts as a barrier between any semen (cum) or pre-seminal fluid (pre-cum), vaginal fluid, rectal fluids/anal mucous or oral fluid (saliva), which is how many STIs are passed on.

Download the cards, cut them out and provide a set for each young person. The task is to arrange the cards into the correct order to show how to correctly use an external condom.

Check the expiry date of the condom.
Check there are no tears or rips in the packet.
If using a water-based lubricant, put a small amount onto the tip of the penis or sex toy.
Move the condom to one side of the pack and carefully tear the pack open.

Remove the condom and check it is the correct way round, roll it onto the erect penis or sex toy.
If using a water-based lubricant, put this all over the condom.
After sex, carefully remove the condom.
Throw it away in a bin.

Ask the young people to do the same for internal condoms (sometimes referred to as a female condom).

Internal condoms act in the same way as the external condom, except they are inserted into the vagina or anus.

Download the cards, cut them out, mix them up and give sets of cards to each young person. They must arrange the cards in the correct order to show how to safely use an internal condom.

Put lubricant on the outside of the closed end.
Find a comfortable position – stand with one foot resting on a chair, sit on the edge of a chair, lie down or squat.
Squeeze together the sides of the inner ring at the closed end of the condom and insert it into the vagina or anus. (Insert into the vagina like a tampon, pushing the inner ring as far as it can go, until it reaches the cervix.)
After sex, gently pull the condom out of the vagina or anus.
Dispose of it in a bin.

Sexually transmitted infections including genital herpes, chlamydia, syphilis, gonorrhoea and hepatitis can also be passed on through unprotected oral sex.

A dam is a thin square piece of latex which is placed over the anal or vaginal areas during oral sex and can be used to protect against STIs. Dams can be purchased from chemists and sexual health and family planning clinics.

ACTIVITY: DILEMMA: WHAT COULD YOU DO?

Ask the young people to consider the following scenarios:

- Seth and Amy had sexual intercourse but unfortunately the condom had split.
- Jo and Adam did not plan to have sex, but then they did. Jo was waiting for Adam to mention condoms but he didn't and they didn't either and so sex happened without condom use.

Discuss in a group what options are open to young people in these situations. If the condom was torn or broken during sexual activity or if no condom was used, there are a number of things young people can do to reduce the risk of STIs and unplanned pregnancy.

If the young person was not using another form of contraception, they could get emergency contraception. They should also get an STI test. If required, they should take any preventive medicine.

Post-exposure prophylaxis or PEP is a course of anti-HIV medication. It could prevent a person from developing the HIV infection if they have been exposed to the virus. A person may have been exposed to HIV if they have:

- had unprotected sex (without using a condom)
- had sex with someone with HIV and the condom broke
- been injured with an HIV-infected needle.

ACTIVITY: EMERGENCY CONTRACEPTION FACTS

Test your young people's knowledge with these true or false questions.

True or false?
Emergency contraception only works the morning after.

False: Many people believe that emergency contraception can only be taken in the 24 hours after sex. But this is not true. Some types can be taken up to five days after sex has taken place.

There are two types of emergency contraception.

True: There are emergency contraceptive pills and the intrauterine device or IUD (a copper coil). There are two types of pill; one which needs to be taken within 72 hours of unprotected sex and one which is effective for up to five days after. The IUD needs to be inserted into the uterus within five days in order to be effective.

Emergency contraception works every time.

False: Unfortunately, this is not true. Emergency contraceptive pills are effective only if taken before ovulation occurs and so it would depend on a woman's menstrual cycle. The sooner emergency contraception is taken the more effective it will be. The IUD is the most effective form of emergency contraception.

You can only get emergency contraception from your doctor.

False: In the UK, emergency contraception is available for free from GP surgeries, sexual health services, NHS walk-in centres and, if required, A&E departments in hospitals. Many pharmacies also have emergency contraception available, which you have to pay for (this would also require a short consultation with a pharmacist).

Taking emergency contraception too often has a negative impact on fertility.

False: There is no evidence to suggest that taking emergency contraception regularly will have a negative effect on fertility. Being proactive about sexual health may be a better way of managing the risk of unplanned pregnancy and so considering an alternative form of contraception and using condoms is advised.

REPRODUCTIVE CHOICES

Introducing the topic: Reproductive choice is not only about avoiding unplanned pregnancy, but also about having wanted children. It includes a person's choices around pregnancy prevention, protection from STIs and HIV, termination of an unplanned pregnancy, having a healthy pregnancy and baby, fostering and adoption, and intervention to influence fertility.

There is a lot of medical terminology used when discussing reproductive choices and fertility. It can be helpful to understand these terms in order to be informed.

ACTIVITY: UNDERSTANDING THE REPRODUCTIVE TERMS

Download and cut out the reproductive terms and description cards, mixing them up. Provide each young person or group with a set of the cards and task them with correctly matching the term to the correct description.

Ejaculation	Semen is the fluid produced by the male sexual organs to protect and carry sperm. The word describes when the fluid comes from the penis.
Insemination	Treatment that involves directly inserting sperm into a woman's womb.
Menstrual cycle	The monthly changes that occur in the female reproductive system (specifically, the uterus and ovaries) which make pregnancy possible.
Menopause	The time when menstrual periods stop permanently, and women are no longer able to have children. For most women, this happens at about 51+ years.
Ovulation	The release of the mature egg, sometimes called the ovum, from the ovaries.

Ovaries	Two oval-shaped organs that produce female eggs.
Testicles (also called testes or balls)	Oval-shaped organs that sit in a sac that hangs behind the penis. Their main job is to make and store sperm.
Infertility	A problem of the reproductive system which can affect men and women. Defined as when a person has not been able to achieve a pregnancy after 12 months or more of regular sex without contraception. Nine to fifteen per cent of couples will have fertility problems.
Fertile window	A specific time in a women's menstrual cycle when it's possible to get pregnant.
Miscarriage	The loss of a pregnancy during the first 23 weeks. The main sign of this happening is vaginal bleeding, which may be followed by cramping and pain in the lower abdomen.
Abortion or termination of pregnancy	Where pregnancy is ended either by taking medicines or having a surgical procedure.
Adoption	Making the choice to deliver the baby and the baby is looked after by another person or couple, who become the legal parents.

PREGNANCY CHOICES

Introducing the topic: Before beginning the topic, revisit the working agreement or ground rules ensuring that you have a discussion which covers confidentiality and respect. The topic of pregnancy choices can be highly emotive and we can never be sure what experience the young people we are working with have had. The session should never be a place for debate, but should focus on providing factual rather than value-based information. Adoption can be an emotive topic and again, you may be unaware of young people's personal circumstances and experiences. Ensure all of the options are presented in an equal and unbiased way.

ACTIVITY: IN HER SHOES

Explain to the young people how someone might know that they are pregnant. There is guidance below to help with this. A missed or late period is often the first sign of pregnancy; this is easier to spot for people with a regular cycle. If a young person has recently had unprotected sexual intercourse they should take a test. This would be best carried out at a young people's sexual health clinic or service where the person would also receive information, advice and guidance from the worker about their positive or negative result.

In the result of a positive pregnancy test a young person would then need to make a decision from the three following options: abortion, adoption or becoming a parent.

Task the young people to think more carefully about the options available to a young person who discovers they are pregnant. They could create a table like the one below to list the things a young person may consider which would help her make the right choice for her.

Abortion	Adoption	Becoming a parent

ACTIVITY: YOUNG PEOPLE'S SEXUAL HEALTH SERVICES

In the UK, around one in three women will have an abortion during their lifetime (My Body My Life n.d.). Abortions are legal when carried out up to 24 weeks into the pregnancy. Two doctors need to agree for the procedure to go ahead. Abortions are safe but there are lots of myths people have heard about what they are, how they happen and about young people's rights.

Brook is a young people's sexual health service where young people can visit and get a pregnancy test, see a nurse and be referred for a termination of pregnancy.

Task the young people to visit the Brook website and to write down what information they can find about abortion. (You could also use an alternative website of a young person's service which is local to you or the NHS website.)

Have the young people feed back their findings by creating a mind map of information covering:

- early medical abortions, medical abortions, suction and vacuum, surgical evacuation
- what happens after 24 weeks
- whether parents have to be told
- whether you have to stay in hospital.

ACTIVITY: FATHERS' RIGHTS

Facilitate a discussion around the rights of men/the father when it comes to pregnancy choices. Does having no legal right mean there is no responsibility? Men have the right to avoid conceiving unplanned pregnancies either by choosing not to have sex or to use condoms.

BECOMING A TEEN PARENT

Introducing the topic: Teenage parents will face similar ups and downs to parents of any age, although parenting as a teenager can have added challenges such as continuing education, adjusting to living at home with a baby, and managing new and existing family relationships. Some young parents also feel judged and that there is stigma attached to becoming a young mum or dad. Outcomes for children of teenage parents can be impacted, but with support, many teenage parents overcome these challenges and the parents and children grow up to reach their full potential.

ACTIVITY: A DAY IN THE LIFE OF

Have the young people map out all of the things that they do in a week, the times they wake up, when they do school and classes, time they spend with friends, quiet times, when they eat, sleep, do homework. Encourage them to complete the diary with as much detail as possible.

Once this is complete, ask them to think about the care needs of a new baby. Consider things like what time they wake up, eat, sleep. A typical baby aged three months may have a schedule like this:

7:00 am	Wake and feed	6:30 pm	Awake and play
8:30 am	Feed and nap	7:30 pm	Bedtime routine – bath
11:30 am	Feed and nap	8:00 pm	Feed and bedtime
2:30 pm	Feed and nap	11:00 pm	Top-up feed
5:30 pm	Feed and nap		

How does the schedule of care for a new baby impact the life of the teen? Use the talking points to explore this further.

TALKING POINTS

- How does taking care of a baby fit with the typical day of a teen?
- What extra support would young people need to be able to continue to do all of the things they did before becoming a parent?
- For someone wanting to have children, what could be the ideal age or time for them to start a family?
- What factors should be considered when making choices about starting a family?

Exploring parenting and choices can raise lots of questions for teens about their future, plans, goals, dreams and aspirations. I have found this next activity to be one which can be supportive of this and works well when exploring these topics.

ACTIVITY: BY 100 TIMELINE

Have the young people create a timeline starting from the age they are now until they are 100. Ask them to think about all of the things they might want to achieve in this time. Would they like to finish school, go to college, pass their driving test, go to university, go to a club, get the job of their dreams, get a dog, run a marathon, swim with dolphins, write a book, buy a house, set up a charity, travel the world, marry, adopt, retire and so on? Ask the young people to map on a timeline the age by which they would like to achieve these.

Next, ask the young people to take a step back and look at the things they have listed. Do these require them to have achieved something or reached a milestone before they can do these things? For example, if they said buy a house, would they need a deposit?

Using the timeline, the young person can now look at setting themselves some short-term and long-term goals. Short-term goals should be achievable within a number of months, or within a few years. Long-term goals are bigger ambitions which may also have many stages and require more long-term forward planning. There is a lot of psychological research that supports goal-setting as a great tool for building self-esteem.

And there are proven health outcomes from positive esteem, such as better resilience, less risk-taking, and informed decision-making.

▼ Goal planner

Start date: . . . .

End date: . . . .

My short-term goal/s:

My long-term goal/s:

My strategy:

To do list:

My progress:

◆ Chapter 8 ◆

Health Education

INTRODUCTION

From 2020, alongside the introduction of compulsory RSE, health education became a mandatory subject in all English schools. The guidance means that all pupils will now be taught about good physical and mental health, with the aim to help young people grow into healthy and happy adults.

The learning outcomes suggested as part of health education ensure a programme or work will include mental resilience, confidence building and developing the skills required to know when you need to seek help.

Topics such as cancer awareness and the benefits of a healthier lifestyle, and its impact on preventing ill-health, will also be covered, which sit nicely alongside the topics featured in the new reformed relationships and sex education in secondary schools.

The health education programme now also incorporates many of today's relevant and key issues, which many of the young people we work with will experience. Online safety and topics such as cyberbullying and sexting have also been included.

The programme for secondary-aged young people leads on from the primary school programme which delivers age-appropriate relationships education, featuring healthy friendships and family relationships, as well as puberty and menstrual wellbeing topics.

As well as informing young people and providing them with what they need to know about these topics, health education should also provide opportunities to develop skills and explore values and attitudes. The activities in this section aim to support young people to develop their confidence and resilience and to feel empowered.

PERIOD TALK

Before compulsory health education, many schools did not deliver period education outside what was taught in science. Discussions around period management options, period poverty or menstrual issues were not included, and many young people were only taught the basics, focusing on a 28-day cycle.

Reports from a number of charities also discovered that the lack of education meant that many girls getting their period for the first time didn't know what it was and what was happening to them (Plan UK 2018); 48 per cent of girls described feeling embarrassed about their periods, with the figure rising to 56 per cent for 14-year-olds (Plan UK 2017). The same study asked a group of girls and young women if they had felt prepared for their first period, and, shockingly, all of the participants taking part said no. Words and phrases used by the female participants to describe starting their periods included 'scared', 'horrible', 'no clue what was happening', 'I thought I was going to die', 'shocked', 'embarrassed', 'unprepared'.

It seems crazy that periods, which can be experienced by half of the population and which are an everyday part of healthy lives, are still so taboo. To this day, I still discover a huge knowledge gap, and many misunderstandings when training teachers, alongside an uncomfortableness to talk openly about the topic with the young people they teach.

Knowing your body is one of the topics covered in this book. It introduces a collection of fun and engaging activities which are integral to learning about periods. It is also a necessity for contraception, fertility, consent, body autonomy and pleasure as part of relationships education.

CANCER AWARENESS

Another topic introduced into health education is young people learning about cancer, particularly cancers which may impact them and where self-examination and screening are required. From Year 10 onwards, young people will learn about testicular cancer, breast self-examination and cervical cancer screening. Research carried out by the cancer charity Eve Appeal (2018) found that two-thirds of UK parents supported cancer awareness being taught in schools, many of them admitting the topic was something they felt uncomfortable to talk about at home.

SINGLE GENDER VS MIXED GROUPS

I would encourage all genders to have the opportunity to learn together and to learn about each other. This can help to reduce the stigma which surrounds many of the relationships, sex and health education topics. It can also help young people to develop their empathy skills, when given the opportunity to learn about the differences and similarities of the issues many girls and boys face.

Single-gendered groups, in my experience, have always been positive too. Providing a space for this as well as mixed group learning would be great if timings allow for that.

PUBERTY

Introducing the topic: Puberty is the phase when physical changes take place in the body signifying the transition from childhood to adulthood. The body starts producing chemicals called hormones that cause changes to happen in various parts of the body.

ACTIVITY: PUBERTY QUIZ

Test the young people's knowledge and help them to learn more about puberty using these questions and answers.

1. Do boys and girls start puberty at the same age?

Answer: Girls usually start puberty earlier than boys, this can be around 8–13 years and 10–15 years for boys.

2. During puberty, are the changes in the body caused by hormones?

Answer: Yes! Boys make a hormone called testosterone (formed in the testes). Girls make oestrogen and progesterone (made in the ovaries).

3. Does the brain influence the changes which happen during puberty?

Answer: Yes. One or two years before puberty a part of the brain called the pituitary secretes a hormone which tells the ovaries and testes to start producing the sex hormones.

4. During puberty will both boys and girls start to see changes in their body shape?

Answer: Yes, this is one of the earliest changes. Girls start to develop breasts, may gain weight and grow taller. Boys grow taller and more muscular and get hairier.

5. Are acne and pimples common during puberty?

Answer: Yes. Due to the increase in hormones the skin becomes oilier. This may be more severe in some people than others. Cleansing with water and soap helps. If you are worried about your skin, you can also speak to a doctor or nurse.

6. Is it normal to have mood swings during puberty?

Answer: Yes, it is normal to feel upset, sad and maybe a bit self-conscious. It can help to talk to a trusted adult, sharing worries and talking about feelings.

7. Can hormonal changes cause sexual feelings?

Answer: Yes. The hormones can make you feel attracted to someone you like or admire. It is also normal for people to want to explore, touch and learn more about their body. It is normal if you do, and normal if you don't.

8. During puberty, do boys and girls sweat more?

Answer: Yes. It's quite usual to sweat more. This can cause an unpleasant body odour and so it will become important to keep your body clean, use an antiperspirant, take regular baths and wear clean clothes.

9. Is it normal for boys to have nocturnal emissions or wet dreams?

Answer: Yes, wet dreams can happen. As the penis and testicles develop and hormones are released, semen can come from the end of the penis during the night and you may wake up with wet underwear.

10. At what age does puberty end?

Answer: 17–19 years. The stage of puberty continues until around 17 years for girls and 19 years for boys.

ACTIVITY: PUBERTY IN PICTURES

Using the downloadable page which shows the outline of a body, young people can be encouraged to write about, draw and label the changes that happen to children and young people during puberty. Get them to also consider the thoughts, feelings and anything else they associate with this time or change. You can get really creative and draw a life-size person, creating a display in the school or community centre.

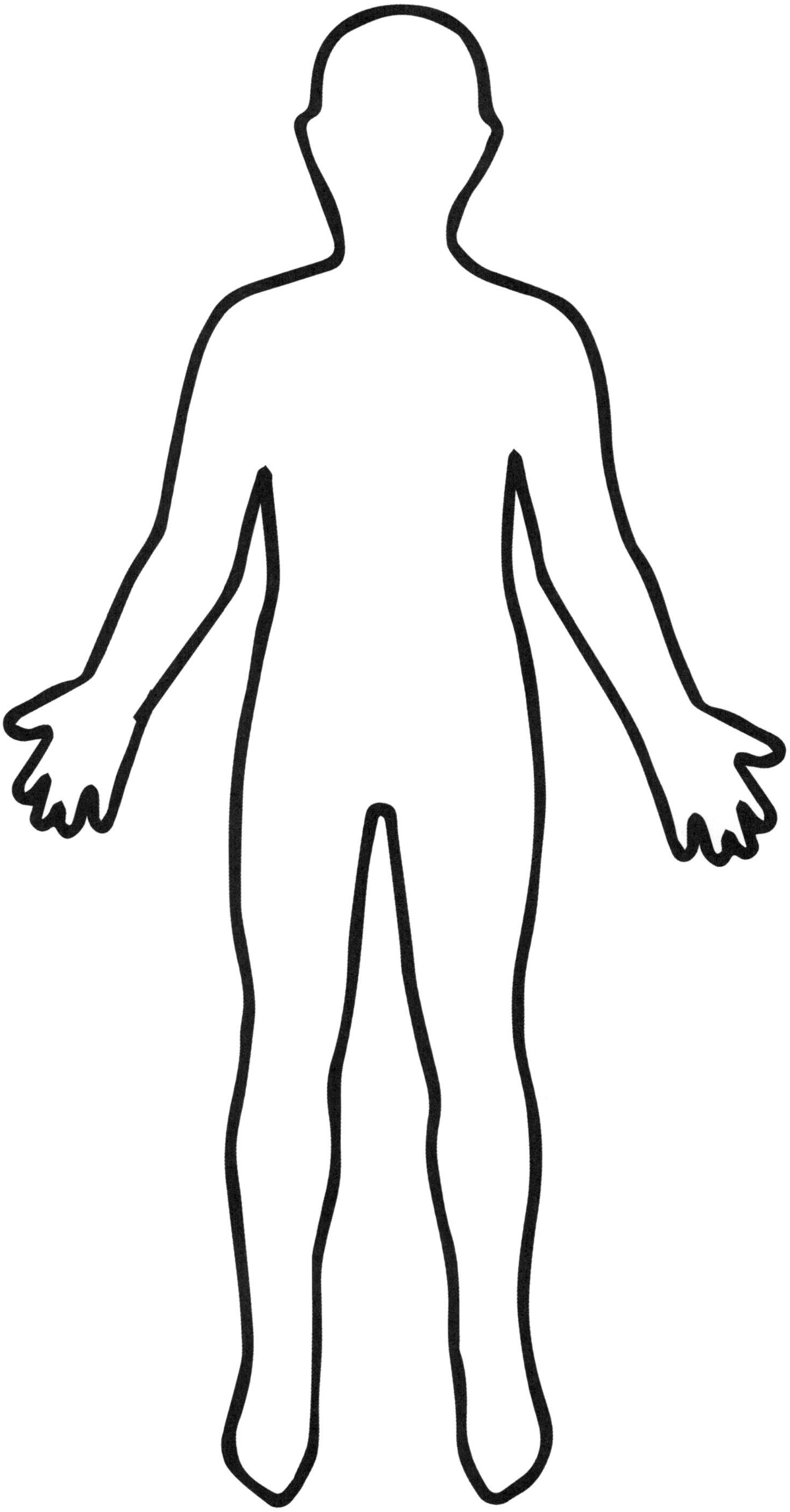

ACTIVITY: THE PUBERTY BOX

Create a puberty box. This is a great visual tool that can be used to support discussions about puberty, body image, pressure, personal hygiene and beauty myths.

Here are some ideas of what you could include in your puberty box:

- Antiperspirant deodorants
- Perfumed body spray
- Body wash, soap, face wash, hand wash, hand sanitiser, and shampoo
- Boxers and briefs
- My first bra example
- Period products including: pad, pad with wings, panty-liner, tampon with cardboard applicator, tampon with plastic applicator, non-applicator tampon, menstrual cup, period absorbent underwear
- Razors/hair removal products (men's and women's variety), including razor, hair removal creams, wax strips, shaving foam
- Spot creams
- Feminine hygiene washes and products
- Make-up

It is important to become familiar with the contents of your puberty box and to consider the possible discussion points for each of the items before sharing them with young people.

The puberty box creates a great learning environment to discuss and explore beauty standards and ideals and body image pressures. Sexism is often a topic of discussion too, encouraged by the packaging and branding and price differences often found.

A great activity which assists the learning from the puberty box is to get a blank pack of playing cards and have the young people create an information card for each of the products.

ASK A TRICKY QUESTION

Introducing the topic: It is great practice to provide opportunities where young people can ask or submit anonymous questions or concerns. Make sure you let young people know in advance that these opportunities to ask questions are going to be available so they can think about what they might want to say. Promote the use of the anonymous questions opportunity in other topics workshops and sessions too.

ACTIVITY: ONLINE SURVEYS AND QUESTIONNAIRES

Google forms, Microsoft forms and SurveyMonkey all allow you to create surveys in which the young people can remain anonymous. Create an 'ask a tricky question' survey which invites young people to submit their own questions or share any worries they may have.

Explore with them what is meant by a tricky question: this could be a question which they feel too embarrassed to ask out loud, or one which they couldn't get the answer to from somewhere else. It could be one which they feel uncomfortable seeking the answer to online. Collect the questions submitted and use these to plan workshops and activities.

ACTIVITY: ANONYMOUS QUESTION BOX

Find a space in your building to place a post box where anonymous questions can be submitted. Think about how often they will be collected, and how they might be answered. What about having an RSE notice board with frequently asked questions which are updated each month.

ACTIVITY: EMAIL/SUPPORT

Can you share an email address where young people can submit their questions? You could link this to pastoral staff or team up with a local health and wellbeing team who can offer mentoring and referrals or signposting.

ACTIVITY: WAYS TO RESPOND

You can answer the questions submitted by young people during your RSE workshops and activities, providing the opportunity for a good, old-fashioned, open and honest discussion. This has been and always is my most popular and most enjoyed activity when collecting feedback from young people. It shows that one of the most important factors of RSE is providing a safe space for young people to talk.

Other ideas include: developing and writing a blog on your website, having an agony aunt/ uncle page in the school newspaper, creating a display in the building, producing topic-related advice leaflets and handouts for young people to take home.

ROCK YOUR BODY

Introducing the topic: A painted rock, sometimes called a kindness stone, is a rock or pebble that someone has taken the time to decorate with paint or markers. It often has an inspirational message or picture.

The rocks are then used to spread positivity or raise awareness in the local community. Once the rock is painted and dried, it is left somewhere for another person to find.

ACTIVITY: CREATING THE STONES

To make painted rocks with young people you will need:

- Smooth rocks or stones
- Acrylic paint
- Brushes
- Acrylic paint pens
- Varnish or sealant

Provide a stone or rock for each young person and task them to create a Rock Your Body stone. The stone should include a positive message for young people growing up and experiencing puberty, which will encourage them to love who they are and to not conform to any body image pressures. Messages, such as 'Your body your rules', 'All bodies are good bodies', 'Be you not them', can be shared to spark creativity.

Once painted, the young people will need to decide where they will leave the stones ready for others to find.

You could create a hashtag or an @ which can encourage those who find the stone to visit the hashtag or account and share the stone's journey with the young people. This can be really interesting, fun and encouraging.

KNOW YOUR BODY

Introducing the topic: Knowing the correct terminology, names and functions for the reproductive body parts is an important part of health education, and relationships and sex education too. Many families often use slang terms for private body parts, teaching these to children as they grow up, but recent studies have shown that this can have a negative effect on young people and adults. It can lead to them feeling embarrassed to talk about their bodies with their partners, hindering confident communication about boundaries and contraception, and evidence suggests it can stop adults and young people from seeking information and health advice when they have worries.

When young people know the correct names for their body parts, it can make learning about lots of body and health topics easier and it can support young people to develop the great communication skills needed to ask questions and seek advice when they need to.

ACTIVITY: SLANG GLOSSARY

What do we mean by private parts? Why are these parts of our body known as private? Can you link the discussion to any laws, including sexual harassment or consent?

Have the young people create a list covering what are the most commonly used slang terms for the private parts of the male and female body – it can be helpful to revisit ground rules before doing this and agree any terms which would be unacceptable and why.

Once you have two lists, one for male and one for female, compare the two. What can be identified from the types of names that are used, and how can these terms support and encourage gender stereotypes, sexism and body image pressures?

To extend the activity you could go on to create a glossary for the key words.

ACTIVITY: IT'S SCIENTIFIC!

Use the downloadable worksheets to check if the young people can label the male and female reproductive system and genitals, using only medical and scientific terms. Follow this up with a discussion using the talking points.

TALKING POINTS

- Why do you think so many people, including adults, feel embarrassed or ashamed to use the correct terminology for the reproductive system and genitals?
- Why is it important that we work hard to overcome this?

Can you label these diagrams, using only medical and scientific terms for the male and female reproductive systems and genitals?

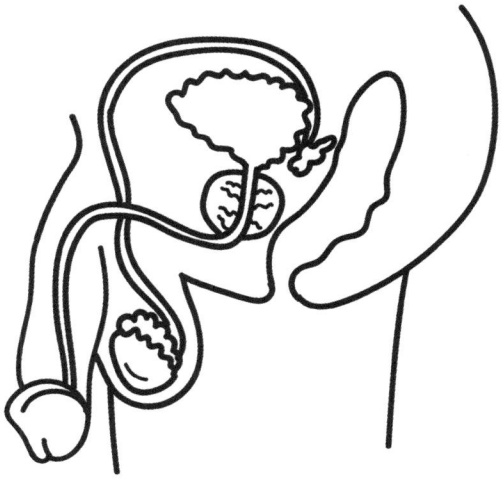

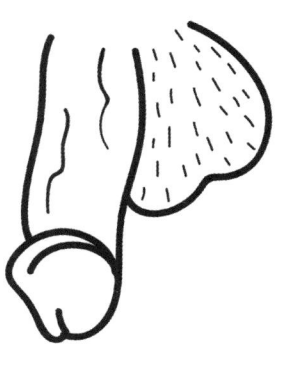

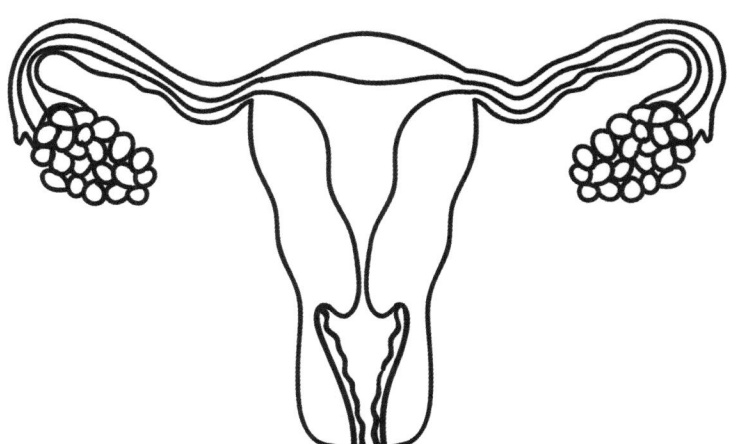

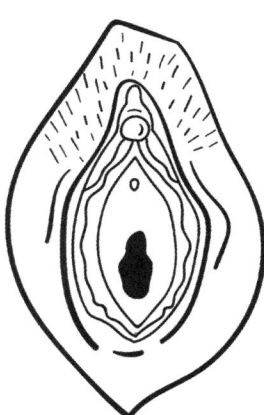

Answers

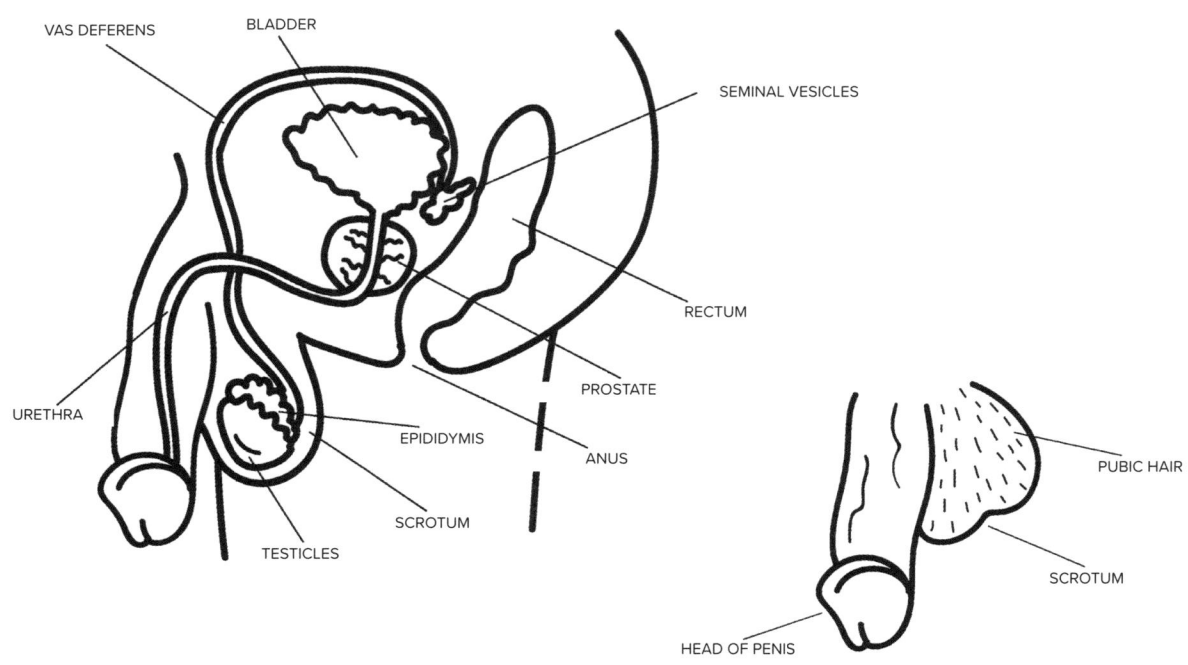

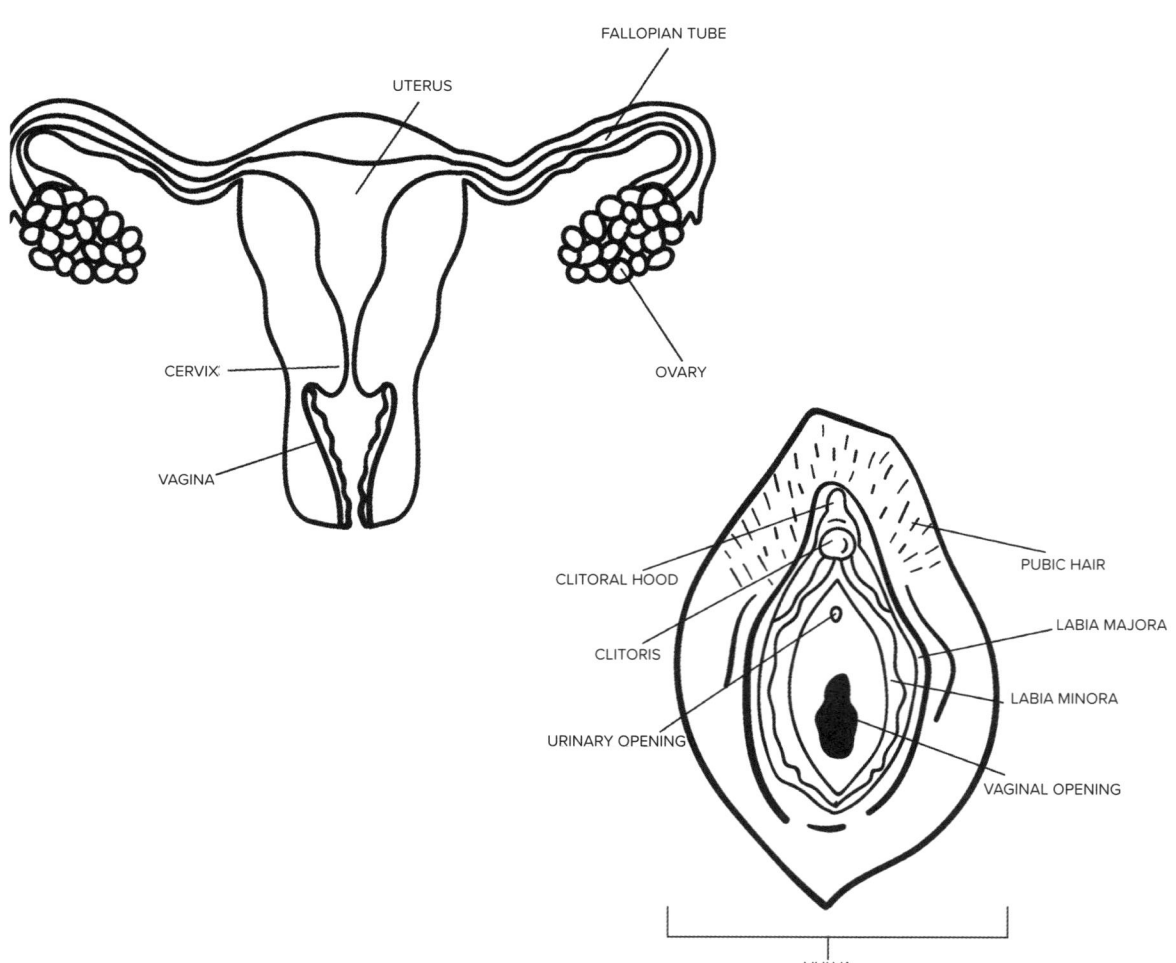

ACTIVITY: WHAT DO I DO?

Following on from the last activity, this extension card sorting game can help young people understand different functions of the reproductive system. Download and print the page, cut up the words and descriptions, and ask the young people to match the correct term to the correct description. The answers are given below:

Penis	Part of the male reproductive system. Also used to pass urine (wee).
Testis/testicle	The two male sex organs that hang behind the penis, which produce sperm and male sex hormones (testosterone).
Scrotum	The sac that hangs behind the penis containing the testicles.
Vas deferens	The thin muscular tube that transports the sperm from the epididymis to the urethra.
Urethra	The tube that carries urine from the bladder to the outside of the body – it runs down the middle of the penis.
Prostate gland	Supplies fluid for the sperm during ejaculation.
Epididymis	A tube where sperm is stored.
Seminal vesicle	Located at the base of the bladder, these secrete a fluid (semen) that nourishes the sperm.
Fallopian tube	The tube joining the ovary to the womb along which eggs travel.
Ovary	Part of the female reproductive system that produces and stores eggs in women and girls at puberty.
Womb (uterus)	The place inside a woman where a baby develops. Also, the lining of this is shed during a girl's period.
Vagina	The entrance between a girl or woman's legs that leads to the womb.
Cervix	The entrance to the womb at the top of the vagina.

Male reproductive system cards

Penis
Testis/testicle
Scrotum
Vas deferens
Urethra
Prostate gland
Epididymis
Seminal vesicle

Part of the male reproductive system. Also used to pass urine (wee).
The two male sex organs that hang behind the penis, which produce sperm and male sex hormones (testosterone).
The sac that hangs behind the penis containing the testicles.
The thin muscular tube that transports the sperm from the epididymis to the urethra.
The tube that carries urine from the bladder to the outside of the body – it runs down the middle of the penis.
Supplies fluid for the sperm during ejaculation.
A tube where sperm is stored.
Located at the base of the bladder, these secrete a fluid (semen) that nourishes the sperm.

Female reproductive system cards

Fallopian tube
Ovary
Womb (uterus)
Vagina
Cervix

The tube joining the ovary to the womb along which eggs travel.
Part of the female reproductive system that produces and stores eggs in women and girls at puberty.
The place inside a woman where a baby develops. Also, the lining of this is shed during a girl's period.
The entrance between a girl or woman's legs that leads to the womb.
The entrance to the womb at the top of the vagina.

PERIODS

ACTIVITY: TRUE OR FALSE

The average person who menstruates will have around 400–500 periods in their lifetime. Yet there is still so much information around the topic of periods that is misunderstood. Young people may hear a lot of myths about menstruation. Use this true or false quiz to introduce the group to these fun facts about periods.

Print the downloadable quiz and hand out one per person. Allow time for the group to complete the quiz, reading each statement and answering either true, false or not sure. Use the answer sheet on the next page to provide the correct information.

 Write true, false or not sure in the box.

The average age that girls start their periods by is 12 years old.	
A period happens when the lining of the womb comes away and comes out of the vagina.	
When a girl has a period, she loses about 250ml of blood.	
A girl has a period around every seven days.	
A period can last from 14 to 28 days.	
Periods are mostly unpleasant and painful.	
A girl may feel emotional and sensitive before and during her period.	
When a girl is having her period, she should not play sports or go swimming.	
Women have periods until the menopause which happens on average when women reach the age of 35.	
Boys have periods too.	
A girl starts her periods because her ovaries have started to release eggs.	
When a girl is on her period, she has two period management choices: tampons and menstrual cups.	
If a girl has not started menstruating by the time she is 14 there is a fertility issue.	

ANSWERS AND TALKING POINTS: TRUE OR FALSE ACTIVITY

The age that most girls start their periods by is 12 years old.	False: The age can be anytime between around 10 and 15, although some girls may be younger or older.
A period happens when the lining of the womb comes away and comes out of the vagina.	True: The lining of uterus breaks down and sheds, resulting in period blood leaving from the vaginal opening.
When a girl has a period, she loses about 250ml of blood.	False: Most girls will lose less than 80ml of blood. Some woman may have heavy menstrual bleeding; they lose more blood and may have periods that last longer than seven days.
A girl has a period around every seven days.	False: A period cycle is around every 28 days although teenagers may find they can be irregular and happen less often.
A period can last from 14 to 28 days.	False: An average period can last between one and seven days.
Periods for some girls can be unpleasant and painful.	True: Some girls will suffer from heavier and painful periods. If this happens, they can speak to a nurse who can advise them.
A girl may feel emotional and sensitive before and during her period.	True: The emotional changes that happen are caused by fluctuating hormone levels.
When a girl is having her period, she should not play sports or go swimming.	False: Girls can do all of the things they can when they are not on their period. Finding the right period management product can help.
Women have periods until the menopause which happens on average when women reach the age of 35.	False: The menopause, when a woman stops having periods, happens around the age of 51.
Boys have periods too.	Language and terminology is changing to become more inclusive to all genders and non-binary people. Many places use the terms person with a vagina when talking about periods to be supportive and inclusive to trans people.
A girl starts her periods because her ovaries have started to release eggs.	True: Ovulation is when an egg is released from one of the ovaries during a menstrual cycle. The egg travels down the fallopian tubes and the womb prepares for implantation. You can only get pregnant if the egg is fertilized by sperm.

When a girl is on her period, she has two period management choices: tampons and menstrual cups.	False: There are many options available to manage the flow from the vagina which happens during periods. Other options include pads and period underwear.
If a girl has not started menstruating by the time she is 14 there is a fertility issue.	False: Some girls don't start their periods until they are 15 or older. Once a woman has a regular cycle, and then it becomes less regular, infrequent or absent this could indicate an issue with ovulation. Heavier or more painful periods could be a sign of endometriosis.

PERIOD TABOOS

Introducing the topic: A menstrual taboo is any social taboo concerned with menstruation. Many ancient cultures and texts considered menstruation unclean or embarrassing. These beliefs date back thousands of years but still influence cultural stigmas around discussing and caring for menstrual needs in today's society.

Did you know that in some parts of the world women are made to live in menstrual huts during their periods and for up to two weeks after giving birth? Taboos around periods still exist in areas where sanitation and period management products are still underdeveloped.

Other stigmas about periods include girls who live in all male households or with male parent/s. These girls may think they cannot talk openly to their families about their periods, the idea being that men don't understand and don't want to hear about it. This is often reinforced in the media through advertising and also in comedy.

ACTIVITY: TALK TABOOS

Have the young people brainstorm all of the words that come to mind when thinking about and talking about periods. This can include slang terms too. Write these on the board.

Common answers may include: embarrassing, annoying, painful, smell, uncomfortable. You may find that many of the words are negative: time of the month, lady problems.

Discuss with the young people why periods are thought of in this way. Refer back to the ancient taboos, and linking this to the taboos we see in today society.

Some examples of this could include discussing whether educating boys, young men and fathers about periods is a good idea.

Here are some other discussion points you could introduce.

Girls who start their periods when they are younger also face shame and embarrassment. Many start their periods before they have been taught about them and are often scared. They may be the only one of their friends to have started and find that other friends don't understand, and many realize that schools and other places where they go are not designed for young women having periods. Many primary school toilets don't have facilities for sanitary disposal and so when a girl starts her period, she may be asked to use the staff or disabled toilet. Why might this be difficult for her?

Many transgender and non-binary young people feel excluded when periods are talked about as being a 'woman thing'; similarly, when we associate having a period as a sign of being a woman, we also exclude the women who don't have periods for a number of different reasons.

How can we make period education and period management more inclusive?

Period poverty is an issue facing many girls, both from across the world and in the UK. Period poverty is a term to describe when a person is unable to access sanitary products often due to financial constraints.

A report by Plan International UK (Plan UK 2017) found that one in ten girls can't afford to buy menstrual products, and one in seven have at some point struggled to afford them.

The same report found that:

- 49 per cent of girls have missed an entire day of school because of their period
- 59 per cent of these girls have made up a lie or an alternative excuse to avoid going to school
- 137,700 children in the UK miss school each year because of period poverty.

ACTIVITY: PRESENTING PERIODS

Task the young people to create a presentation which aims to normalize speaking about periods. They can design the presentation for one of these audiences:

- Dads
- Primary-aged children
- Teenagers.

MANAGING PERIODS

Introducing the topic: There are many period management options for young people that are designed to absorb the menstrual blood and prevent staining on clothes. There are also menstrual cups and period pants.

Gather some samples of different the different types of pads and tampons available for the next activity.

ACTIVITY: PERIOD MANAGEMENT

Use the period management samples you have and pass these around so that each young person can take a closer look at them during the discussion.

Menstrual pads have a sticky adhesive strip on the back, which is used to secure them in the underwear, absorbing the period blood as it leaves the vagina. Tampons are inserted into the vagina and absorb the period blood before it leaves the body. To explore this further you could:

- use a diagram or model to show how the tampon fits inside the body
- put a tampon in a glass of water to show how it absorbs and holds fluid
- demonstrate how a pad is placed into the underwear and how it can be disposed of.

Some young people choose to use environmentally friendly products that can be reused. There are environmentally friendly pads and tampons available. Talk with the young people about these ethical choices.

Another option is a menstrual cup. Show a menstrual cup and demonstrate how these are used. (You can find some great videos on brand websites; many also offer a free demonstration model for educators.)

 To conclude, use the downloadable worksheet to summarise the discussion points.

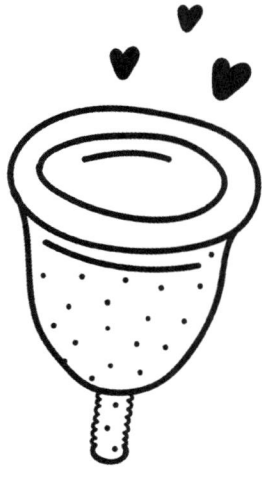

Menstrual cups are reusable and are made of silicone. The cup is inserted into the vagina and it collects menstrual blood. You use your fingers to remove this and empty the contents down the toilet, rinse the cup with water and place it back inside the vagina.

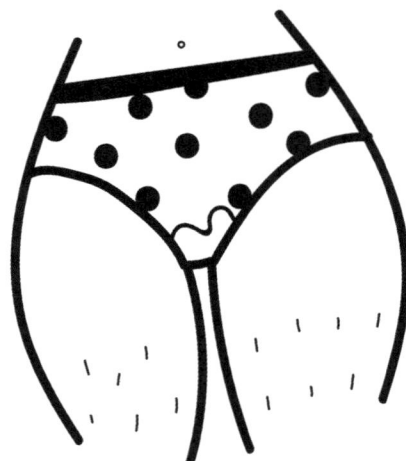

Periods pants are a reusable underwear which can be worn all day and protect by absorbing the period blood. They have to be rinsed in cold water after use and can then be washed in the laundry. They are available in a range of styles and shapes.

Fill in the blanks with the appropriate word from the box.

Pads

Pads come in different . . . .
(for example, regular, long), thicknesses (for example, maxi, super, mini, night time), and styles (for example, with or without . . . ., with or without deodorant).

Pads are placed in the . . . . to absorb menstrual blood.

Pads need to be changed every . . . . hours or more often if the period is heavy.

Pads can be worn . . . .

If a pad is unavailable, you can make an alternative by folding up . . . .

Tampons

Tampons are inserted into the . . . . to catch menstrual blood before it leaves the body.

Tampons come in a variety of sizes and . . . . (for example, regular, super); some come with plastic or cardboard applicators to help with insertion.

Some people never use tampons, some use them for . . . . or certain activities, and some use them as their choice to manage periods.

Tampons should be changed every . . . . hours or more often if needed.

Tampons should not be worn for longer than eight hours and should not be worn overnight due to the risk of a rare infection called . . . .

Tampons cannot get lost in the body since the . . . . stops them from going into the uterus.

Used tampons can be wrapped in toilet paper and put in the bin or flushed.

Answers: Pads

underwear	toilet paper	sizes	three to four	wings	overnight

Answers: Tampons

vagina	absorbencies	swimming	four to six	toxic shock syndrome	cervix

ACTIVITY: NAME THE PRICE

Bloody Good Period is a charity that provides menstrual supplies to food banks and community groups. In a recent article on its website it was estimated that the average lifetime cost of having a period is about £4800 (Lee 2018). Create price cards for each of the menstrual products. Calculate these for the year. Ask the young people to guess which price card is for which product.

Here are some average costs: menstrual cup £20 (lasts ten years); reusable pads, 15 cost around £100 and last around five years.

Following on from this you could also suggest that the young people design an advertising poster for one of the menstrual products they have learned about. Remind them to think about its unique selling points and what makes it a good choice to use. Get them to consider what other important information would be relevant to let somebody know who was looking to buy period products.

Encourage them to think about how they can also make their adverts inclusive and how they can use their advertising poster to challenge taboos and end stigma.

BODY HEALTH CHECK

Introducing the topic: With all these changes happening to young people and their bodies, it is important that they begin to take care of themselves. Self-care is an important part of health education.

Here are some things young people should start to think about:

- Eating well and exercise
- Personal hygiene
- Mental wellbeing.

Eating well and exercise: What's good? A well-balanced diet, including lots of fresh fruit and veg. Drinking plenty of water. Exercising! If young people don't enjoy sport, they could try dancing at home, riding a bike to school, taking their dog for a walk. It's easier to get exercise if people choose something to do that they enjoy.

What's not so great? Fatty foods, fried foods and sugary foods (e.g. pastries, biscuits, chips, sweets). Diet fads, or social media health trends should be avoided. They don't work.

Personal hygiene: Once young people reach puberty, they may find that they sweat more. This is normal! Sweat does not have much of a smell but bacteria which live on the skin can create a smell called body odour or BO. To avoid body odour, young people need to wash their bodies daily, especially the underarm area, using mild soap and warm water. They should also change and wash their clothes often. An underarm deodorant may be useful too.

Mental wellbeing: It is just as important to take care of mental wellbeing as it is physical health. During puberty, hormones can make young people feel giddy and excited or moody and emotional; everyone will have their ups and downs. Some top tips for positive mental wellbeing are to get enough sleep, and take time to relax. Remind young people to be kind to themselves. Sometimes they need some extra help to look after their mental health. Suggest that if they are feeling this way, they should speak to a trusted adult.

There are so many activity ideas which can help young people to support self-care. For example, you could:

- use the puberty box to explore and discuss different aspects of personal hygiene
- taste test fruit and vegetables, or create a healthy breakfast recipe
- teach some relaxation techniques and breathing exercises
- make a face mask made using natural products.

Get the young people to write down all the things they already do and the things they could do to take better care of themselves, and share their ideas with each other. Part of this could also be to list the names of trusted adults and places they can go for help and support with any worries they have.

TESTICULAR CANCER AND TESTICULAR SELF-EXAMINATION (TSE)

Introducing the topic: Before teaching about testicular cancer awareness, it would be helpful to revisit learning from the Know Your Body activities which covered the naming of the parts of the male reproductive system and genitalia. This is an important aspect of the topic, as the terminology and functions will help young people better understand the information which will be explored here.

This topic includes lots of information; it can be used to create a digital presentation to assist with the discussions you will have. There are also some differentiated activities below that can be used if the young people have already completed the Know Your Body task.

ACTIVITY: DRAW SOMETHING

Have the young people use a large sheet of paper to draw, label, correctly name and describe the functions of the male reproductive organs and genitals.

ACTIVITY: PUT A PIN IN IT

As a group, draw or display a large diagram of the male reproductive anatomy and make cards with the different body parts on them. Ask the young people to take it in turns to try and place the name card on the correct body part. To make this more fun you could add blindfolds.

ACTIVITY: MALE MODELS

Using soft dough, clay or other model-making materials, such as pipe cleaners, tissue paper, loo roles and ping pong balls, task the young people to make the male reproductive system in three dimensions.

TALKING POINTS

These talking points are a great way to inform young people and help dispel any myths they may have about their bodies. Discussing this information with young people can help develop their confidence to seek help about any body worries they may have.

The penis

Penises vary in size and appearance. There is a wide, natural variation in the size of adult penises, but when erect, they are mostly similar in size. (Share some penis facts, if you have any – depending on the age and stage of the group.)

- What's the average penis size?

There are no average length figures for teenagers because people grow at different rates. For men, it is 5–7 inches, smallest recorded 2, largest 13.

The foreskin is a fold of skin which covers the tip of the penis (glans). It is very important to keep the area beneath it clean. The foreskin should be pushed back daily and the glans gently washed.

Sometimes the foreskin is removed surgically at birth. This operation is known as circumcision and is performed by some groups as part of their cultural and religious beliefs. Some young men may notice that the foreskin is tight, which can cause infection and make it painful when passing urine. If this happens, the young person needs to speak to their GP who can prescribe creams and may arrange for the young man to be circumcised for medical reasons.

The testes

During puberty, there is a change in the functioning of the testicles (testes), which is caused by the body's production of the male hormone testosterone. This means that the testicles begin to produce sperm.

Sperm are shaped like tadpoles, with 'tails' that enable them to move. Sperm are so tiny that they can only be seen under a microscope.

- How many sperm can a man produce?

The average male will produce roughly 525 billion sperm cells over a lifetime. A healthy adult male can release between 40 million and 1.2 billion sperm cells in a single ejaculation.

Testicles need to be kept cool to support sperm development. This is why they hang outside the body in a sac (bag) called the scrotum.

It is quite normal for one testicle (testis) to be larger or to hang lower than the other.

At birth, some boys may have experienced what is called an 'undescended testicle' where one or both testicles fail to move down into the scrotum. This is usually corrected after birth.

Testicles that have moved down into the scrotum will sometimes pull back into the body, for instance in cold water. This is quite normal. They will eventually move back into place on their own. Any concerns young people have about differences in the testicles can be talked over with a doctor.

- Why should young men check their balls?
- Have you heard of testicular cancer?
- What do you already know?

Testicular cancer facts

Testicular cancer is the most common cancer in young men – and the good news is that it's a cancer which is extremely curable.

If a young man discovers a lump or swelling, or a heavy feeling in his testicles, he should be encouraged to get this checked out. Most lumps and bumps don't turn out to be cancer.

The age range most at risk of testicular cancer is young men aged from 15 to 30 years.

Once a young man has reached puberty, it is a good idea for him to begin to regularly check the size and shape of his testicles. It is perfectly normal for one of the testicles to be bigger than the other.

The purpose of the testicle checks, also known as a testicular self-examination or TSE, is for young men to get to know the size, shape and texture of their testicles and to understand what is right and 'normal' for them. A good time to do this is when taking a shower.

If a young man checks his body regularly, and gets to know himself, he will find it easier to notice any differences or changes in the testicles, if they occur.

DEMONSTRATING TSE

If possible, share a video which demonstrates TSE. You could also purchase a TSE demonstrator and model how to do this, and you can purchase TSE mini testicle and scrotum models which can be shared to allow young people to have a go at checking the testicles.

ABOUT TESTICULAR CANCER

If a young person has symptoms of testicular cancer, he will be referred to see a specialist who will chat to him and his family and ask lots of questions about their health. It is likely that the specialist will examine the testicles, take a sample of blood and carry out an ultrasound scan of the testicle.

The blood tests are used to identify if a person has high levels of certain chemicals that can be a sign of cancer. The ultrasound scan creates an image for the specialist to see which shows more clearly any lumps or cysts which can be felt – if a clearer image is required, the doctor may carry out an MRI or CT scan.

TREATING TESTICULAR CANCER

The first stage in treating testicular cancer is surgery to remove the testicle. Some young men opt to have a prosthetic testicle fitted in its place, so everything looks like it did before.

If the cancer is found later and is more advanced, a young person might need radiotherapy or chemotherapy, which can stop the cancer returning and target any remaining cancerous cells.

REAL-LIFE STORIES

Bring the lesson to life by including real-life stories of people who have had and have overcome testicular cancer. This can be very empowering and inspiring.

- Why this workshop is so important?

One of the reasons why this workshop is important is because reports show that in general men are less likely than women to seek health advice when they need it, and this can have a real impact on their lives. For example, men are less likely to seek help for gambling issues, alcohol addiction and mental health worries (Mental Health Foundation 2021).

In my own work with boys and young men who are seeking health advice and guidance, I have come across the same trend. My experience of working with groups of young men highlights that many boys and young men are more likely to talk to their friends about a worry or problem they face, and laugh it off rather than talk to a teacher or parent.

- Why do some boys and young men struggle to access health advice, talk about their worries?

ACTIVITY: MAN UP

Ask the young people to:

- think of three words that describe what a man is
- pair up with others in their group to discuss their ideas and write down 10–15 words
- share their ideas with the class.

Discuss the words selected and what they say about being a man:

- Are they a true representation of what it is to be a man?
- Where do we get these ideals/messages from?
- What do our families and the media teach us about what being a man means?
- What happens to men and boys who don't fit these stereotypical ideals?

Introduce and explore the term toxic masculinity. When young men do not conform to the masculine stereotypes, it can lead to gender-based bullying. Young people not living their authentic life leads to unhappiness, worry, stress and engaging in risky behaviours. This is sometimes referred to as toxic masculinity.

Toxic masculinity tells young men that there is one certain way to 'be a man', and this directs how young men look, how they act, how they treat others, and more.

Telling boys and young men to act a certain way can be harmful to young men, their relationships and others. Instead, we should work to ensure people are able to define their own gender.

GIRL TALK

Introducing the topic: Before teaching about young women's health and the female body, it is helpful to revisit learning from the Know Your Body activities which cover the naming of the parts of the female reproductive system and genitalia. There are some differentiated activities below that can be used if the young people have already completed the know your body task.

These activities celebrate the female body and educate young women (and young men), answering many 'am I normal?' questions about the body, growing up and health. These ideas will provide opportunities to explore the topics of body hair, cosmetic surgery, breast cancer awareness (including self-examination), cervical screening and body positivity.

ACTIVITY: ANATOMICALLY CORRECT

Can the young people remember what the female reproductive system looks like? Task them to draw a diagram and use the information from the cards below to help them.

UTERUS/WOMB

The uterus, or womb, is a hollow, pear shaped organ which can expand up to 50cm in length during pregnancy. Two fallopian tubes, one on each side, stretch from the ovaries to the uterus. These tubes carry an egg from one of the ovaries each month, gently moving it along to the uterus.

OVARIES

The ovaries are glands which produce female sex hormones and egg cells (ova). Each ovary is only the size of an almond, but it contains 150,000–200,000 eggs. Every month, from puberty until you reach menopause, one of your ovaries will release one egg (sometimes more, but this is not common). Each egg is around the size of a pinhead. The time when an egg is released is called ovulation.

CERVIX

The bottom of the uterus is connected to the upper part of the vagina by the cervix. The cervix produces mucus. In the days leading up to ovulation, this mucus becomes clear in appearance, and elastic and slippery.

VAGINA

The vagina is a stretchy tube made from muscle. It leads from the cervix to the outside of the body. When you get your period, menstrual blood flows out of your body through the vagina. The vagina is also where a penis enters during sexual intercourse. The vagina is also the birth passage down which a baby travels during childbirth.

VULVA

The vulva is the outside part of a woman's genitals. The vulva includes pubic hair, the inner and outer vaginal lips (labia), the clitoris and the openings of the vagina and urethra. The urethra is the tube which carries urine (wee) away from the bladder. The outer labia are the large fleshy lips of the vulva. The inner labia are the folds of skin that protect the entrance to the vagina and urethra. The inner labia may be covered by the outer labia, but it is also quite normal for them to extend outside. All woman's labia are different in shape and size.

BREASTS

Breasts come in all shapes and sizes. Some young women may worry about the size of theirs and think they are too big or too small. Some young women may worry about the shape and size of their nipples too. There is no right way for breasts to be. It is also completely normal for young women to have one breast hang and be slightly larger in size than the other. Breasts, regardless of their size or shape, are capable of producing breast milk, which is proven to be the healthiest food option for newborn babies.

ACTIVITY: VULVA ART

Using paints, and canvas or soft dough or clay, task the young people to paint or create the female genitalia.

ACTIVITY: WHAT'S ON THE CARD?

Download, print and cut out the cards below, creating several sets. Break the young people into groups and provide them with a set of cards. Each young person takes a card and when it is their turn, they must describe to the rest of the group what is on their card without saying what it is. They can act out the word, describe it, but they cannot spell it out, make a rhyme of it, or give the letter it begins with.

Ovaries	Fallopian Tubes
Uterus	Cervix
Vagina	Urethra
Vulva	Anus
Breast	Nipple
Body Hair	Period
Egg	Hormones

ACTIVITY: TAKE SIDES

Divide the room into two sides and when young people enter get them to take a seat on whichever side of the room they choose. (There should be equal numbers on either side.)

Once everyone is seated and has a side, tell the young people that one side will be the 'for' side, and the other will be the 'against' side.

Explain that it does not matter if the young person is actually for or against the given topic. The idea is that they will be able to think about and generate a presentation which will put forward why they are for or against, but to do this they may have to think about what someone who does agree or disagree might think or say about the topic.

The topic up for debate is female body hair, and the statement the class will debate is 'Women should remove their body hair'. It is important to cover ground rules and explain that the topic may be sensitive to some and that we must remain respectful. Allow students time to think about what their groups for and against arguments will be and provide them with large paper to be able to create a presentation. Encourage them to use facts and not just opinions. They can also look at advertising and media messages which could be helpful to both sides.

ACTIVITY: MY BODY MY BUSINESS

Some mature women choose to shave or wax the hair under their arms, on their legs or in the pubic area. There is no health-related reason for doing this. Young women should not feel persuaded by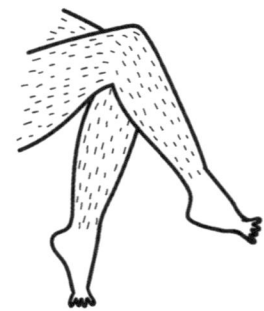

the media stereotypes of female beauty or by peer pressure. If a young woman chooses to remove or not to remove her body hair it should be her choice.

Gather samples of both male and female related hair removal products, such as shaving products and hair removal creams, and prepare a variety of advertising examples to share. Look at the branding of the products, the slogans, tag lines, the way emotive pulls are used. Discuss what messages we receive about body hair from the beauty industry and advertising.

TALKING POINTS

- Do both men and women face the same pressures when it comes to body hair and hair removal?
- How can the beauty industry and media do better to remove the beauty pressures on women and men?

WOMEN'S BREAST CANCER AWARENESS

Introducing the topic: Although breast cancer is very rare for young women, it is one of the most common types of cancer. Breast Cancer Now (2021) estimates that one in seven women in the UK will develop the disease during their lifetime. By increasing awareness and teaching about self-examination, it is hoped that both women and men will become more alert to the signs and symptoms, spotting any changes sooner and speaking to a health professional earlier, when breast cancer is more easily treatable.

These activities will raise awareness and help lower the risk even more. The idea behind these body positive activities is to encourage young people to develop new and healthy habits that support them to look after their own health and bodies.

Providing young people with the knowledge and the skills required to safely carry out a breast self-check will help young women and young men to understand what is normal for them, and spot any changes sooner.

WHAT IS BREAST SELF-EXAMINATION (BSE)?

BSE is when a person carries out a visual and physical check, looking and feeling for any changes in the breasts and underarm area. BSE is something which should be practised as part of self-care and looking after our own health. Breast care also includes women being invited to attend to have a mammogram, an x-ray that can spot cancers when they're too small to see or feel. All women from the age of 50, who are registered with a GP, are automatically invited for breast cancer screening every three years.

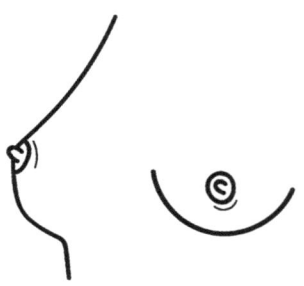

WHEN SHOULD BSE BE DONE?

By doing BSE regularly, a person will get to know how their breasts normally feel and look so that they are able to detect any changes more easily. People can begin practising breast self-examination once their body has developed.

Breast self-examination can be performed every month to help people become familiar with how their breasts usually look and feel so that they can notice any changes from what is their normal. The best time to do BSE is a few days after a period has ended when the breasts are less tender or swollen than they may be during the menstrual cycle.

HOW TO DO BSE

A mirror is useful as the breasts can be seen clearly. Each breast should be checked for anything unusual. The skin should be checked for puckering, dimpling or scaliness. Any discharge from the nipples should be noticed.

The person should place one hand behind the head to stretch the chest muscles slightly. The pads of the fingers of the other hand can be used to check the breast and the surrounding area, including the underarm, pressing down firmly. The idea is to check for any unusual lumps or bumps under the skin. Some people prefer to do this in the shower, as the soap and water can help the fingers glide over the skin more easily. Time should be taken to check and feel the whole area, and this should be repeated on the other side.

If a person sees or feels any changes, these should be checked with a doctor or nurse. Changes in the breasts may include:

- signs of a lump
- a discharge from the nipple
- swelling of the breast
- skin irritation, such as redness, thickening, or dimpling of the overlying skin
- swollen lymph nodes, which are in the armpit
- any pain or redness of the nipple.

It can be very frightening to see or feel something different while performing a breast self-examination. But it is important not to panic. Sometimes, the lumpiness may be due to hormonal changes or something else, and most breast lumps are benign, which means they are non-cancerous.

Once the demonstration has been carried out, allow for questions and then repeat the demonstration again, this time tasking the group to also take scribble notes.

Scribble notes are the use of illustrations, boxes, headings and words which are scribbled or sketched to create a visual picture of the information and discussion. They are a fun way for young people to retain information and boost memory.

ACTIVITY: SCRIBBLE NOTES

Provide young people with a piece of paper and pens for notetaking.

Using a BSE model, if you have one, demonstrate to the group of young people how to carry out a breast self-examination. If you don't have a model, you can use the palm of your hand to demonstrate.

You can also find a great range of videos and resources online produced by cancer awareness charities, such as Coppafeel!, which are aimed at young people.

For the first demonstration ask the students to pay their full attention.

Once the demonstration has been carried out, allow for questions and then repeat the demonstration again, this time tasking the group to also take scribble notes.

Scribble notes are the use of illustrations, boxes, heading and words which are scribbled or sketched to create a visual picture of the information and discussion. They are a fun way for young people to retain information and boost memory.

ALL BODIES ARE GOOD BODIES

Introducing the topic: Body image concerns are seen to impact children from a young age and cause worry for both boys and girls, although many studies suggest the impact is greater for young women.

In a UK study by Be Real (2017), 79 per cent of 11–16-year-olds said that how they look is important to them. The study also found that 52 per cent of young people said they often worry about the way they look.

In young people, body dissatisfaction has been linked to risk-taking behaviours and mental health problems. The 2020 Girls' Attitudes (Girlguiding 2020) Survey found that 80 per cent of girls and young women aged 11–21 have thought about changing their appearance. The study highlighted how young women feel it can be challenging to relax and enjoy themselves and some explained their worries about being themselves, and how their confidence drops as they get older.

INTRODUCING BODY POSITIVITY

Body positivity is the idea that all people are entitled to have a positive body image, regardless of how they fit society's and popular culture's ideals around body shape, size and appearance.

Here are some aims linked to the body positivity movement:

- Promoting the acceptance of all bodies – all bodies are good bodies!
- Supporting young people to build their self-confidence and acceptance of their own bodies.
- Speaking out about the unrealistic body standards we see.
- Challenging society's views around body image.

Body positivity also includes challenging beauty and body ideals based on race, gender, sexuality and disability.

Providing opportunities for young people to build their body confidence and self-esteem can have positive outcomes, and research has found that young people with greater body appreciation are less likely to diet or use alcohol or cigarettes (Andrew, Tiggemann & Clark 2016).

Promoting body positivity also includes teaching young people about how popular media messages contribute to the relationship that people have with their bodies, including how they feel about fashion, diet, nutrition, fitness, identity, health and self-care.

ACTIVITY: BODY POSITIVE AFFIRMATIONS

In this activity, young people will train their brains to hear and believe the kind things they have to say about themselves. By saying body positive affirmations, they'll be speaking and hearing the things they need to hear to help build their confidence.

Start by getting them to list all of the things their body can do and achieve that they are thankful for.

From the list, they then choose five things which they will create an affirmation for. An affirmation is a positive statement that can help to overcome any negative self-thoughts. Saying the affirmations reminds the brain to feel good and release its feel-good hormones.

Some examples of positive self-affirmations are:

- I am a good role model; I am positive and my positive outlook inspires others.
- I am not afraid to take risks. I am brave and I go for it. I aim to live my best life.
- I will not put myself in a situation that is not respecting me. I make decisions that will make me feel good.

Distribute some black postcard-sized pieces of card and pens and task the young people to get creative and design a set of three positive affirmation postcards.

ACTIVITY: COMPLIMENT CARDS

Complimenting someone when they least expect it can put a smile on their face (and ours, because doing good deeds can make us feel good too).

In this activity, the young people will spread feelings of confidence, resilience, empowerment and body positivity by sending someone they know a compliment card.

Task the young people to use one of the postcards designed in the last activity, write a kind message on it and send it to someone they know.

ACTIVITY: MOOD BOARD

The media can influence the way young people feel and think about themselves. Evidence suggests that often this can be a negative impact, highlighting imperfections and shaping body ideals. Young people can counteract these negative influences by becoming more aware and critically thinking about and questioning the things they see, hear and read in the media. They can also counteract the negative images by surrounding their spaces with positive media influences. For this activity, young people will create a body positive mood board. There are two ways you can do this activity. One is using print media, such as magazines, advertising and newspapers, cutting out words and images to create a positive message; the second way is using Pinterest or similar to create a board online which can then also include media files.

ACTIVITY: BODY POSITIVI-TEE

If we are looking to raise awareness of body positivity then wearing a custom t-shirt to share these messages could be a perfect place to start.

Before working on the digital designs with young people, use a t-shirt template and get them to think about their ideas, why they want to create it, what aspect they want to raise awareness of, and who will be wearing their t-shirt.

Then task the young people to think of a punchy slogan that would grab the attention of others and get their message across. After creating their design on paper, they can then draw this onto a plain t-shirt using fabric markers or paints or design it online using a platform like Canva and get the finalized t-shirt printed. You could host a competition getting everyone in the community involved.

FEELINGS AND EMOTIONS

Introducing the topic: Understanding our emotions is an important part of emotional literacy, which is crucial for healthy relationships. Becoming aware of what we are feeling can help us to deal with life stresses and also supports us to enjoy and make the most of good times.

Check-ins are a great way to enable young people to develop the skills to talk about and start to express how they are feeling. You can introduce check-in activities at the beginning of an RSE session.

Here are five quick and fun feelings and emotions check-in ideas:

CHECK-IN 1: THE WEATHER REPORT

Ask the young people: If your mood was today's weather, what weather would it be?

- Thunderstorm = angry
- Sunny = happy
- Rain = upset
- Hail = hurt
- Rainbow = excited

Give everyone a chance to think and choose, then facilitate their answers, sharing with the whole group.

It can also be fun to visualize the task by creating a weather map and making the different weathers; the young people can then take their chosen weather and place it on the map, saying how they feel.

CHECK-IN 2: DRAW HOW YOU FEEL

Ask the young people how their mood is today. Using a range of colours, shapes, swirls, arrows, scribbles, dots (anything goes), the young people then draw how they are feeling today/this week or about the task, session in hand.

You can have the group draw on one large sheet of paper on a shared smartboard, or they could create individual drawings for themselves. You can facilitate a discussion and young people can choose to explain their feelings, or not.

CHECK-IN 3: THE YOUNG PEOPLE'S PLAYLIST

Ask the young people: If their current mood could be represented by a song, what song would it be? Whether it be the lyrics, or the sound, task young people to choose a song which represents how they feel about a given situation. For example, if they're having an amazing day, it could be 'Happy' by Pharrell Williams. Give everyone a chance to think, then have everyone share their song with the group. You could create the playlist on a popular music app and play it during the session.

CHECK-IN 4: TOPS AND PANTS

To make this check-in visual, you can use card to cut out tops (t-shirt templates) and pants (trouser templates) to write on. Ask the young people to think about their 'tops and pants' of the day or week/weekend. Tops represent the best thing that has happened to them during this time, and the pants represent the worst thing that has happened to them.

CHECK-IN 5: START, STOP, CONTINUE

Task the young people to think of their 'start, stop, and continue' goals of the day or week. The start is something they are going to start doing – a change they are going to make; their stop is something that they would like to stop doing; and the continue is a good thing they did during the day or week that they are going to keep doing.

Give everyone a chance to think, then go around the circle and have everyone share with the group.

ACTIVITY: MAPPING YOUR FEELINGS

Most of us will have felt 'butterflies' in our tummy, or had 'cold feet', a 'gut reaction' or a 'shiver down our spine'. Every day we use words and saying like these to describe how emotions make our body feel. When we take risk, or feel unsafe, our bodies tell us through physical sensations that something is wrong. We may also get these feelings when we take healthy risks and so it is good practice to explore the differences between the two.

Using the outline of the body, task the young people to write, draw or label where and how our bodies work with us to show us how we feel. Explore how we should respond to these warning signs and also consider situations when it is okay to push through these feelings and possible situations and when it is important to take note and listen.

ACTIVITY: MANAGING YOUR EMOTIONS

Anger

Fear

Anticipation

Surprise

Joy

Sadness

Trust

Stress

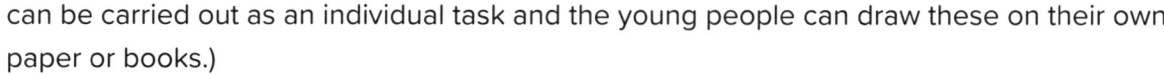

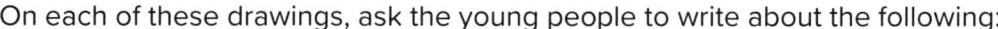

Anger is a normal and healthy feeling we will have all experienced at some point in our lives. Part of our emotional literacy is to learn how to manage our anger, so we can talk about frustration or unhappiness without making a situation worse. Sometimes we get angry in the moment, and other times we may have bottled things up for a long time.

Using a board or a piece of large display paper, draw an image of a bottle, a flame and a balloon. These should be large enough to include comments written by young people. (If preferred, the activity can be carried out as an individual task and the young people can draw these on their own paper or books.)

On each of these drawings, ask the young people to write about the following:

- In the bottle: a situation which they have bottled up.
- In the flame: how it feels when they bottle things up.
- In the balloon: a solution which could help them let these feelings go.

ACTIVITY: COOL DOWN

One easy way to calm down our body's responses to anger and to help reduce any stress is to slow and deepen our breathing. Try this quick breathing exercise with young people, developing their skills to use this technique whenever they need to cool down.

You can make this more fun by using chocolates too (Maltesers work well). Find a quiet space where young people will be able to lay down and relax, guide them through the steps:

1. Lie on your back, relax your muscles, lower the shoulders and allow the body to flop.
2. Take a Malteser or similar and place this over closed lips.
3. Start by breathing slowly into your nose and then out through your mouth.
4. Breathe deeply from your belly rather than your chest.
5. When blowing out through your mouth, try to carefully blow the Malteser, balancing it.
6. Repeat until you feel better (then eat the chocolate).

ACTIVITY: CHIN UP

If there is one sure fire way to help everyone feel better it's laughing.

Laughter can decrease stress hormones and trigger the release of endorphins, which are the body's natural feel-good chemicals.

A chin face, sometimes referred to as a chinikin, chinhead, chinman or chinmonster, is a performance, usually of a comical nature, involving someone's chin. It can be a great visual tool and a fun activity to bring about laugher and lift up spirits.

Get the young people working in pairs and give out some googly eyes; you can also draw a tie or dickie bow on a sheet of paper.

Once the young people have decorated their chins, they can work in small groups and hang upside down and sing, or lipsync, to their favourite songs. If you are able to, you can make funny videos of the chinikins and make a whole group montage, watching it back together and laughing out loud.

ACTIVITY: COLOUR ME CALM

Can you guess how many emotions a human can experience? According to psychologists it's around 34,000 (Karimova 2021). Working as a whole group, create a list of as many emotions as you can think of.

Once complete, share the emotions wheel (this can be easily found on the internet). The emotions wheel was developed by American psychologist Dr Robert Plutchik, who proposed that there are eight primary emotions, which serve as the foundation for all others. Plutchik's theory defines the eight basic emotions as:

1. Fear – feeling of being afraid, frightened, scared.
2. Anger – feeling angry. A stronger word for anger is rage.
3. Sadness – feeling sad. Other words are sorrow, grief (a stronger feeling, for example, when someone has died).
4. Joy – feeling happy. Other words are happiness, gladness.
5. Disgust – feeling something is wrong or nasty. Strong disapproval.
6. Surprise – being unprepared for something.
7. Trust – a positive emotion; admiration is stronger; acceptance is weaker.
8. Anticipation – in the sense of looking forward positively to something which is going to happen. Expectation is more neutral.

These eight basic emotions were also assigned to a specific colour, with the intensity of colour increasing with the strength of the emotion.

Spend some time looking at the wheel with the group. Are there any emotions on the wheel which did not appear on the emotion list the group created?

Pair up the young people to work together and provide each pair with an emotion that is relevant and relatable to young people (you can take these from the list which they created earlier). The task is to write a definition or description of the emotion. Each pair can read these out to the other pairs and see if they can identify the emotion from the description they gave.

ACTIVITY: FEELING AND EMOTIONS COLOUR SWATCH

Task the young people to choose five of the emotions which best represent how they feel most often, and on an ongoing basis.

They must then choose a colour that they think best applies to and represents each of their chosen emotions. The young people will then be tasked to design and create their own colour swatch bookmark using the emotions and colours they have chosen.

The bookmark can be used to share with each other how they are feeling on a particular day, about an activity and so on. They make a great resource to have on the desk to let others know how we are feeling each day so others can then respond accordingly.

ACTIVITY: SPELL YOUR NAME CHALLENGE

Start with a whole group challenge and have the class complete an A–Z of positive words, writing down as many positive words as they can think of for each letter of the alphabet. It could be helpful to set a time for this to be complete.

Following this, the young people use the A–Z to create an illustrated poster which spells their name with a positive word for each letter.

Positive words starting with the letter A

absolutely | adorable | accepted | acclaimed | accomplish | accomplishment | achievement | action | active | admire | adventure | affirm | amazing | attractive | awesome | able | accepting | appreciative | assertive | aware | authentic | accountable | acknowledging | adventurous | adaptable | agile | alert | affectionate | ambitious | amazing | attentive | authentic | animated | adored | amusing | advantageous | assured | articulate | astounding | approachable |

Positive words starting with the letter B

beaming | beautiful | believable | bliss | bountiful | brave | bubbly | blessed | blooming | balanced | blossoming | brilliant | best | bold | bright | belonging | breathtaking | blazing | beauty

Positive words starting with the letter C

calm | celebrated | certain | champion | charming | cheery | classic | clean | composed | cool | creative | cute | caring | charming | capable | creative | comforting | cuddly | cheerful | committed | curious | compassionate | connected | courageous | competent | consistent | contribution | courtesy | cooperation | closeness | carefree | credible | clever | compassionate | considerate | cautious | captivating | confident | courteous | curious | constructive

Positive words starting with the letter D

dazzling | delightful | distinguished | divine | delicious | dreamy | daring | decisive | delighted | dynamic | delicate | deserving | decent | desire | devotion | dignity | dazzled | devoted | drive | diversity | dependability | dedication | discovery | deep | determined | diligent | dedicated | detailed | discreet | dependable | diplomatic

Positive words starting with the letter E

effective | efficient | effortless | electrifying | elegant | enchanting | encouraging | endorsed | energetic | energized | engaging | ethical | excellent | exciting | exquisite | empathic | educated | empowered | encouraging | energizing | excited | experience | expertise | eager | elevate | evolve | expression | empowering | exhilarating | enthusiastic | ecstatic | equality | exemplary | extraordinary | effortless | easy going | entertaining | endearing | enterprising

Positive words starting with the letter F

fabulous | fair | fantastic | free | fresh | flourishing | friendly | fun | funny | flowing | family | focused | fulfilled | forgiving | fascinating | fancy | fearless | fit | frank

Positive words starting with the letter G

generous | genius | genuine | giving | glamorous | glowing | good | graceful | great | growing | giddy | giving | great | gorgeous | grounded | grateful | gentle

Positive words starting with the letter H

happy | healthy | heart-warming | honest | honourable | humble | hopeful | hero | holy | helpful | holistic | hot | humorous | handsome | hard-working | hilarious

Positive words starting with the letter I

ideal | imaginative | impressive | independent | innovative | instinctive | intuitive | intelligent | inspiration | interesting | inquisitive | impartial

Positive words starting with the letter J

jovial | jubilant | joyful | jolly

Positive words starting with the letter K

kind | kindness | knowledgeable | keen

Positive words starting with the letter L

legendary | lively | lovely | lucky | leader | loving | loyal

Positive words starting with the letter M

meaningful | motivating | mindful | memorable | mesmerizing | majestic | methodical | magnetic | modest

Positive words starting with the letter N

natural | nice | nurturing | noble | neat

Positive words starting with the letter O

open | optimistic | outstanding | outgoing | organized | original | open-minded | objective | observant | outspoken

Positive words starting with the letter P

positive | phenomenal | pleasant | powerful | prepared | productive | proud | peace | prosperity | patient | playful | polite

Positive words starting with the letter Q

quality | quiet | quirky | queen

Positive words starting with the letter R

reassuring | refined | refreshing | relaxed | respectful | resourceful | responsible | renewed | resilient | resolute | reflective

Positive words starting with the letter S

safe | skillful | sparkling | special | spirited | successful | sunny | super | superb | supporting | surprising | selfless | sincere | sympathetic | strong

Positive words starting with the letter T

terrific | thorough | thriving | top | tranquil | trusting | truthful | thankful | thankfulness | tolerant | thoughtful

Positive words starting with the letter U

uplifting | unconditional | upbeat | upstanding | useful | understanding | unbiased | unique

Positive words starting with the letter V

valued | vibrant | vivacious | valuable | versatile

Positive words starting with the letter W

welcoming | well | wholesome | wonderful | worthy | warm | wholehearted | wise

Positive words starting with the letter X

xoxo

Positive words starting with the letter Y

yes | yummy | yay | you

Positive words starting with the letter Z

zeal | zealous | zest | zing | zestful

ALCOHOL AND DRUGS

Introducing the topic: For many young people, using alcohol, drugs, cigarettes or vaping is considered part of growing up. Many of the young people I work with have given smoking, vaping or alcohol and drugs a try, decided they didn't like the way they made them feel and stopped; however, others continued to use them on a more regular basis, often leading to worrying behaviour and poor health outcomes.

Research about young people and the use of alcohol and drugs, including tobacco, has identified that young people often say they use these substances for the same reasons that adults do: to relax or feel good. Others are curious and want to learn for themselves, and to know what it feels like to get high. And some describe wanting to fit in with their friends – in one workshop I delivered with young people around peer pressure many young people said they would most likely try alcohol and get drunk if they were under pressure from their peers rather than have the confidence to say no.

In communities today, groups of young people may try a number of substances, including cigarettes, vapes, alcohol, inhalants, prescription and over-the-counter medicines, as well as illegal drugs. Statistics show they use alcohol and cannabis more than any other substances (Public Health England 2018).

We know that a young person using alcohol or drugs will often feel the effect of these substances, and using these can lead to a change in how they think and feel, which often affects their decision-making.

Sadly, for some of the young people we work with and support, their alcohol or drug use may turn into an addiction and can lead to health and emotional issues, as well as increase the risk of accidents or crime.

Educators can play a key part in teaching young people about alcohol and drug use by talking openly and honestly about the effects that these can have, and raising awareness of the link between drug use and mental health conditions.

It is also important for young people to be aware of the laws relating to the supply and possession of illegal substances. Alcohol dependency, addiction and increased risk of cancers are also important factors for young people to learn about.

Consideration should be given to young people's lived experiences and it is imperative that educators create a trauma-sensitive, safe and non-judgemental learning space. The aim is to equip young people with the skills, knowledge and attitudes that will enable them to make better and more informed choices regarding tobacco, alcohol and drugs.

The following section will feature activities which can be used with young people to explore the topic of smoking, alcohol and drugs.

ACTIVITY: SMOKING – TRUE OR FALSE

The right side of the room represents true and the left side represents false. Task the young people to listen to the statement being read out and decide which way to go.

Smoke from cigarettes can make people who don't smoke ill.	True
Smoke makes hair and clothing stink.	True
Smoking can affect a person's ability to smell and taste food.	True
One in ten UK cancers are caused by smoking.	False. One in four cancers are caused by smoking.
Smoke can cause red, itchy and watery eyes.	True
Second-hand passive smoking smoke does not affect people's health.	False. Figures show more than 600,000 people in the world, including 165,000 children, die each year from passive smoking (Öberg *et al.* 2011)
E-cigarettes are a safe and risk-free alternative to smoking.	False. There are two concerns with e-cigarettes: device faults and side effects on health.
Cigarettes contain one chemical, called nicotine.	False. Cigarettes contain over 4000 toxic chemicals and around 50 of these cause cancer. The three main toxins are nicotine, carbon monoxide and tar.
It takes about ten seconds for nicotine absorbed into the bloodstream to reach the brain.	True
Smoking is a difficult habit to quit.	True
Nicotine, the chemical found in cigarettes, is an addictive drug.	True. Most smokers do not smoke out of choice, but because they are addicted to nicotine.
Smoking 20 cigarettes a day over one year costs around £1000.	False. It costs around £3000.

ACTIVITY: EVERYBODY DOES IT!

Many assumptions are made about young people around smoking and other topics. In this session you will explore this more. Ask the young people to guess the answers to the following questions:

Question: What percentage of young people aged 11–15 do you think are regular smokers (at least one per week)?

Question: What percentage of young people aged 11–15 do you think have tried smoking at least once?

Answers: In a 2018 survey only 2 per cent of young people said they were regular smokers. In the same survey, 16 per cent of 11–15-year-olds said they had tried smoking at least once (Office for National Statistics 2018).

TALKING POINTS

Knowing that most young people don't smoke, explore how this makes your group of young people feel and think about smoking.

Why do most young people choose not to smoke:

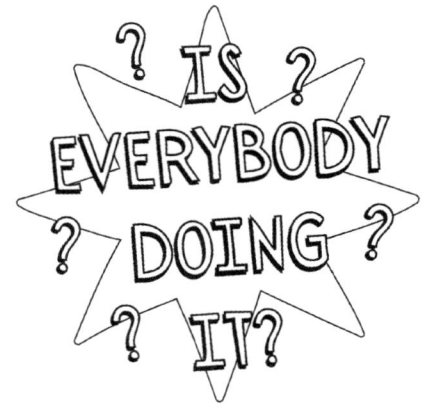

@ TOUGHCOOKIESED

- What are the health reasons?
- What are the social reasons?
- What are the financial reasons?
- What are the legal reasons?

To progress the topic, look further at some of the laws that relate to smoking and tobacco. Ask the young people if there are any that they know of (write down their answers on the board).

Gather and share information about the smoking laws in your area. These could be related to purchasing, sales, and also where smoking is or isn't permitted.

Ask the young people if they are aware of these laws. If they are, do any surprise them?

For the next activity, which aims to help young people think further about how they feel and what they understand about tobacco laws, split the young people into small groups and provide each with a scenario card showing one of the following scenarios for city life. Working in their groups the young people should consider their thoughts as individuals and as a collective, summarizing their ideas and preparing feedback for the whole group.

ACTIVITY: LIFE IN THE BIG SMOKE

Ask the young people to read the scenario card carefully and work with other members of their group to explore what it would be like to live in this city, answering the key questions. Instruct the groups to write their ideas on to flip chart and to prepare to share their ideas with the other groups.

The city of Do-What-You-Like:

You live in the city of Do-What-You-Like. In this city anyone can smoke, no matter what their age, religion or culture. Choosing to smoke is a choice made by each individual. All tobacco, e-cigarettes and vapes are available free of charge. There are no support services for those people who want to quit tobacco. There are no laws about tobacco (e.g. there are no age laws, no smoke-free laws, no manufacturing or advertising laws).

There is, however, tobacco education at school, and information about the impact that smoking can have on your health is freely available. People living in this city have the freedom to make up their own minds about smoking and tobacco.

Questions:

- What would it be like living in this city?
- What health problems do you think might occur?
- What social problems do you think might occur?
- What legal problems do you think might occur?

The city of Just-Say-No:

You live in the city of Just-Say-No. Here smoking is considered to be a poison and is banned for everyone. No tobacco, e-cigarettes or vapes are available in shops or super-markets. Anyone who gets caught smoking is prosecuted. There is no smoking or tobacco education in schools and no health information is shared with the public. The only message shared is that smoking is banned.

Questions:

- What would it be like living in this city?
- What health problems do you think might occur?
- What social problems do you think might occur?
- What legal problems do you think might occur?

ACTIVITY: FEEL THE PRESSURE

Peers can have a massive influence over the way young people act and think, and over the things they do. It can be hard enough for a teen to make a good decision and this can be even more difficult when they are influenced by others. Most friends can be a great influence, for example when they encourage each other to try again or to be kind. But friends and others young people know and associate with can also be a bad influence, for example if they ask them to lie or leave someone out. This is known as peer pressure. Peer pressure can be verbal and non-verbal, and peers often influence each other without saying a word.

Ask the young people to work in small groups, read through the peer pressure scenario cards and consider what the person should/could do in those situations.

They could also use drama and role play. Download the cards, cut them up and give one card per group, asking them to explore the scenario and create the next scene showing what the person should do in that situation.

Thoughts and role plays should then be shared with the wider groups.

PEER PRESSURE SCENARIO 1

One of Mo's friends wants to exclude someone they are friends with from the group because they don't smoke like the rest of the group do. They say he is immature and they don't want to hang around with little kids who aren't willing to take risks. Should Mo exclude the non-smoker friend or maybe encourage him to be more like the others in the group and smoke so they can still hang out?

PEER PRESSURE SCENARIO 2

Rekha is asked by a group of her friends to have a cigarette with them. She doesn't smoke and never has done. They have told her that nobody will find out. Should she give it a try?

PEER PRESSURE SCENARIO 3

Mark is with a group of new friends and trying to impress someone he likes in the group. The conversation turns to smoking and he says he did smoke, but recently quit, even though he has never smoked before. The group, including the person he likes, seem really interested and ask him more questions about quitting, meaning he has to tell more lies. Why doesn't he tell the truth?

PEER PRESSURE SCENARIO 4

Taraji is with a group of friends at the local park. A few of them vape and are doing this in the park. Someone notices an adult walking over and it is a parent of someone in the group. They don't want to be caught with the vape and so ask Taraji to hold it and say it is hers. The adult is friends with Taraji's parents. Should she say it is hers?

PEER PRESSURE SCENARIO 5

Bradley walks into the bathroom at break and sees one of his older friends using an e-cigarette. He tells Bradley to have a try of it too. Bradley doesn't want to but he is being laughed at and his older friend says he is scared and soft. He wants to prove that he is not. Should he have a go, just to prove a point?

> ### PEER PRESSURE SCENARIO 6
>
> Two of Cleo's friends have recently started smoking. Her parents have always been against smoking and feel very strongly about this. But her friends have told her to try, they say it is really good and that her parents are so out of touch and old-fashioned. They make fun of Cleo for listening to her parents. Cleo is not very confident and really enjoys being part of this friendship group. What should she do?

ACTIVITY: TABLE TALK

Explore the topic of smoking and learn more about why young people smoke in this facilitated table talk. Use the table talk discussion cards to get the class group chatting.

Want to make it digital? Connect to a live discussion app and encourage groups or individuals to share their thoughts anonymously from their phones.

Read the card to the group and encourage them to share their thoughts and understanding. Ensure that others in the group put forward their ideas and opinions, and promote respect for each other's differences of opinion.

- Why do young people start smoking?
- Why is it so difficult to give up smoking?
- What do you think of passive smoking?
- Do you think that there should be a total ban on smoking?
- What can be done to stop children smoking?
- Do you think a high tax on cigarettes encourages people to quit smoking?
- Should it be illegal for pregnant women to smoke?
- How are cigarettes advertised in England?
- Should smokers pay higher health costs?
- Does smoking make you seem more sophisticated?
- How is smoking portrayed in the media?

ACTIVITY: DRAW A DRUG USER

Although we have become a society which is much more tolerant of drug use and addiction, there is still a stigma attached to it. We often assume we have a good idea of what a typical drug user or drug addict looks like. These ideas have often been developed from the way people who use drugs have been portrayed in the media, through film, TV shows, music lyrics and newspaper articles. The way users of different drugs are portrayed or whether a person is a high functioning addict or not can lead to the glamourizing of certain drugs and also prevent those with worries about their drug use or addition not seeking help as they don't see themselves as the stereotype.

Challenging stereotypes about drug users and drug addiction can be helpful in tackling the feelings of shame and embarrassment which may prevent people asking for help.

Task the young people to draw a drug addict.

Discuss the drawings in further depth. Did the young people have a particular drug in mind? Often young people drawing an addict will draw a person who uses heroin and not consider other drug addictions, including alcohol.

How many of the drawings are male versus female? There is often a sway to drawing addicts as male even though NHS statistics show that secondary school age boys and girls are equally likely to have taken drugs. However, we then see a change from the age of 16+, with a large proportion of people in treatment settings with substance addiction problems caused by cannabis, alcohol and cocaine being predominantly male (NHS Digital 2018).

Discuss how gender norms and assumed gender roles impact drug use and people seeking help. Males are more likely to engage in risk-taking behaviour – with 'boys will be boys' attitudes – but we also see a more obvious societal stigma and shame around girls and women who take drugs.

Next, think about the cultural connotations. Ask the young people to draw a cannabis addict and to reflect on whether their drawing has changed.

Most people will have formed an idea about what someone who is addicted to drugs looks like. But the truth is, anyone young or old, rich or poor, male or female, gay or straight can become addicted to drugs.

ACTIVITY: CURIOUS MINDS

Task the young people to make a mind map of reasons why young people may experiment with drugs. Examples could include:

- out of curiosity
- because they want to appear older
- to be rebellious
- to be sociable
- because they say it calms nerves or helps cope with stress
- to annoy their parents
- because they are always with people who use drugs
- because their friends pressure them
- because they are unaware of the risk
- because everyone in the family does and their parents don't mind.

Consider with the young people other ways in which someone could appear cool, rebellious, sociable or feel calm and relax their nerves without using substances.

Task the young people to use a free platform like Canva, and design and write a how-to magazine article for teens on one of the following topics:

- How to be cool
- How to be rebellious (and be safe)
- How to be sociable
- How to stay calm.

ACTIVITY: FACT FILES

A fact file is a short report which includes the most important information about a topic.

Fact files are a great way to share facts about a subject. The task can be set as a group work project or individual work. The young people have to work to research their given topic and create their own fact file that will not only help their own learning but also be shared to help educate others.

A fact file can include information such as: slang terms/street names, what the drug is and what is known about its use, the law and class of drug, the risks and ways to reduce harm.

They could also include an illustration or image.

Here is a list of topics to choose from:

Alcohol	Legal highs
Amphetamine	LSD
Anabolic steroids	Magic mushrooms
Cannabis	Nitrous oxide
Cocaine	Tobacco
Ecstasy	

Encourage the use of websites such as DrugWise and Talk to Frank which also give young people a reference point for further information.

SMOKING AND THE BODY

No matter how it is ingested, tobacco is dangerous to our health. There are no substances in any tobacco products that are safe, and most contain acetone, tar, nicotine and carbon monoxide. The substances inhaled through smoking don't just affect the lungs. They can affect the entire body.

Smoking can lead to a variety of ongoing health concerns and complications, as well as long-term effects on the body and how it functions. While smoking can increase the risk of a variety of problems over several years, some of the negative impacts are immediate.

ACTIVITY: WHAT AM I?

Download and print the nine effects cards and nine body cards and cut them out. Task the young people to read the effect and identify the matching body part to help them to understand the symptoms of smoking on the body.

Cigarettes make me less shiny and make me smell.	Cigarette smoke makes me sore and itchy.	Cigarette smoke can cause blockages and develop infections.
Cigarettes can cause damage to me becoming dry, dull in colour and wrinkled.	Cigarettes cause me to stain and I can't take my food as well as others who don't smoke.	Cigarettes make me less fit and it is more difficult for me to breathe.
Cigarettes increase the blood pressure which means I have to beat faster and faster and work much harder.	Cigarettes make me lose my sense of smell and cause damage to my nasal hairs.	Cigarettes leave stains on these and sometimes they shake if I haven't had a cigarette for a while.

Hair	Eyes	Ears
Skin	Mouth	Lungs
Heart	Nose	Hands

Answers

Cigarettes make me less shiny and make me smell. **Hair**	Cigarette smoke makes me sore and itchy. **Eyes**	Cigarette smoke can cause blockages and develop infections. **Ears**
Cigarettes can cause damage to me becoming dry, dull in colour and wrinkled. **Skin**	Cigarettes cause me to stain and I can't take my food as well as others who don't smoke. **Mouth**	Cigarettes make me less fit and it is more difficult for me to breathe. **Lungs**
Cigarettes increase the blood pressure which means I have to beat faster and faster and work much harder. **Heart**	Cigarettes make me lose my sense of smell and cause damage to my nasal hairs. **Nose**	Cigarettes leave stains on these and sometimes they shake if I haven't had a cigarette for a while. **Hands**

ACTIVITY: THE UNIT IS RIGHT

This activity is to help young people understand that alcohol consumption is measured in units, and to raise awareness of the number of units young people who use alcohol may consume. The same activity can also be used to discuss the cost of alcohol and explore the impact this has on young people's attitudes and alcohol choices. With so many different drinks and glass sizes, from shots to pints, it is easy to become confused about how many units are in each drink in relation to the health guidance.

To keep health risks from alcohol to a low level, men and women who consume alcohol are advised not to drink more than 14 units a week on a regular basis.

Knowing about the units can help adults who consume alcohol to stay in control of their drinking.

To make the session more visual and engaging, you could collect a selection of drinks glasses such as pint, half pint, wine glass, shot and cocktail glasses. You could use empty bottles and containers to further explore and consider marketing and advertising laws relating to the branding of alcohol. You could also create a presentation using images of illustrations of the different glass sizes/drink types.

First, ask the young people to guess how many units they assume to be in each of the drinks. Following on from this use the information below to explore the correct answers.

The number of units in each drink is based on the size of the drink, as well as the strength of the alcohol. For example, a pint of strong lager contains three units of alcohol, whereas a pint of low-strength lager has just over two units.

Type of drink	Number of alcohol units
Single small shot of spirits (gin, rum, vodka, whisky, tequila, Sambuca) (25ml, alcohol by volume (ABV) 40%)	1 unit
Large shot of spirits (35ml single measures of spirits)	1.4 units
Alcopop (275ml, ABV 5.5%)	1.5 units
Small glass of red/white/rosé wine (125ml, ABV 12%)	1.5 units
Bottle of lager/beer/cider (330ml, ABV 5%)	1.7 units
Can of lager/beer/cider (440ml, ABV 5.5%)	2 units
Pint of lower-strength lager/beer/cider (ABV 3.6%)	2 units
Standard glass of red/white/rosé wine (175ml, ABV 12%)	3.1 units
Pint of higher-strength lager/beer/cider (ABV 5.2%)	3 units
Large glass of red/white/rosé wine (250ml, ABV 12%)	3 units

ACTIVITY: MISSING WORDS

Alongside government advice regarding alcohol unit consumption, there is also guidance which states when adults should not drink.

Write the missing word sentences on the board. Can the young people guess what the missing word is?

Adults should avoid drinking alcohol	Missing word answer
Before	Driving
Before operating	Machinery
When working at a	Height
When doing . . . . or	Sports or swimming
When taking certain . . . . and	Drugs and medicines
When	Pregnant

ACTIVITY: WORST-CASE SCENARIO/BEST-CASE SCENARIO

One of the effects of drinking too much alcohol, especially for young people, is a change in behaviour.

Break the young people into small groups of about five people, providing each group with paper and pens and one of the alcohol story starters. Have them write this at the top of a piece of paper. As a group, they will now consider what the consequence of this situation could be, creating a story of events which would follow. Encourage the young people to think of the worst-case scenario. The group will pass the piece of paper to each person in the group who will add the next line of the story, leading to a dramatic conclusion.

Here are some alcohol story starters:

- Jonah started vomiting in the street.
- As Keely stood up she couldn't see as well as she usually could; she rubbed her eyes but she still had blurred vision.
- No matter how hard Aleema tried, she felt as if she couldn't stand at all or even walk in a straight line.
- Simon is usually so quiet, the others noticed straight away that he was being louder than normal and saying things he would never normally say.
- Alejandro was so sorry for causing the accident.
- Daisy and Badr were arguing all night and eventually it led to a fight.
- I will never be able to show my face again, I made such a fool of myself.
- Dan woke finding himself in a strange place; he realized he was in hospital.
- This is the worst hangover ever...

Once the groups have completed their stories, ask them to go back to the beginning of the story and, using a different coloured pen, highlight, make notes and identify the key aspects of their story, where they feel something could have been changed or a better decision could have been made which would have reduced any risk, prevented injury or embarrassment and improved the outcomes for those involved.

References

Advertising Standards Authority (2020) *Harm and Offence: Gender Stereotypes Advice*. Available at: www.asa.org.uk/advice-online/harm-and-offence-gender-stereotypes.html.

Andrew, R., Tiggemann, M. & Clark, L. (2016) 'Predictors and health-related outcomes of positive body image in adolescent girls: A prospective study.' *Developmental Psychology*, 52(3), 463–74.

Be Real (2017) *Somebody Like Me: A Report Investigating the Impact of Body Image Anxiety on Young People in the UK*. Available at: www.berealcampaign.co.uk/research/somebody-like-me.

Breast Cancer Now (2021) *Facts and Statistics 2021*. Available at: https://breastcancernow.org/about-us/media/facts-statistics.

Department for Education (2019) *Relationships Education, Relationships and Sex Education (RSE) and Health Education*. Available at: www.gov.uk/government/publications/relationships-education-relationships-and-sex-education-rse-and-health-education.

Department for Education (2020) *Understanding Relationships, Sex and Health Education at your Child's Secondary School – A Guide for Parents*. Available at: https://assets.publishing.service.gov.uk/government/uploads/system/uploads/attachment_data/file/907640/RSE_secondary_schools_guide_for_parents.pdf.

Department for Education (2021) *Sexual Violence and Sexual Harassment Between Children in Schools And Colleges: Advice for Governing Bodies, Proprietors, Headteachers, Principals, Senior Leadership Teams and Designated Safeguarding Leads*. Available at: https://assets.publishing.service.gov.uk/government/uploads/system/uploads/attachment_data/file/1014224/Sexual_violence_and_sexual_harassment_between_children_in_schools_and_colleges.pdf.

Department for Education and Employment (2000) *Sex and Relationship Education Guidance*. London: DfEE Publications.

Equality Act (2010) Available at: www.legislation.gov.uk/ukpga/2010/15/contents.

Eve Appeal (2018) *Put Cancer on the Curriculum*. Available at: https://eveappeal.org.uk/news-awareness/gynae-cancer-awareness-month-2/cancer-and-education.

Fertility Education Initiative (2016) *Fertility Health Summit: Choice not Chance: An Overview of the Meeting*. Available at: www.britishfertilitysociety.org.uk/wp-content/uploads/2016/04/Fertility-Health-Summit-Summary.pdf.

Fowler, F. (2012) *The Concise Oxford Dictionary of Current English*. Oxford: Clarendon Press.

Girlguiding (2020) *Girls' Attitudes Survey: A Snapshot of Girls and Young Women's Lives*. Available at: www.girlguiding.org.uk/girls-making-change/girls-attitudes-survey.

James, E. (2020) *Not Just Collateral Damage: The Hidden Impact of Domestic Abuse on Children*. Ilford: Barnardo's.

Karimova, H. (2021) *The Emotion Wheel: What It Is and How to Use It*. Positivepsychology.com. Available at: https://positivepsychology.com/emotion-wheel.

Katz, A. & El Asam, A. (2020) *Look At Me – Teens, Sexting and Risks Report*. Available at: www.internetmatters.org/wp-content/uploads/2020/06/Internet-Matters-Look-At-Me-Report-1.pdf.

Lee, G. (2018) *Period Poverty is Real. But the Average Woman Isn't Spending £500 a Year on Menstruation.* Channel 4. Available at: www.channel4.com/news/factcheck/period-poverty-is-real-but-the-average-woman-isnt-spending-500-a-year-on-menstruation.

Lewis, R., Tanton, C., Mercer, C.H., Mitchell, C.R. *et al.* (2017) 'Heterosexual practices among young people in Britain: Evidence from three national surveys of sexual attitudes and lifestyles.' *Journal of Adolescent Health*, 61(6), 694–702. doi: 10.1016/j.jadohealth.2017.07.004.

Local Government and Communities Directorate (2016) *Young People's Attitudes to Violence Against Women Report on Findings from the Young People in Scotland Survey 2014.* Available at: www.gov.scot/publications/young-peoples-attitudes-violence-against-women-report-findings-young-people.

Martin, G. (2020) *They Told Me to Change my Clothes. I Changed the Law Instead.* TEDx Warwick TED Conferences. www.youtube.com/watch?v=_K_n-x-W7pY.

Mental Health Foundation (2021) *Men and Mental Health.* Available at: www.mentalhealth.org.uk/a-to-z/m/men-and-mental-health.

Mitchell, H., Allen, H., Sonubi, T., Kuyumdzhieva, G. *et al.* (2020) *Sexually Transmitted Infections and Screening for Chlamydia in England, 2019.* London: Public Health England.

My Body My Life (n.d.) Available at: www.mybody-mylife.org.

Nast, C. (2021) 'How my traumatic experience with upskirting taught me how to be an activist.' *Teen Vogue.* Available at: www.teenvogue.com/story/gina-martin-upskirting-activist.

NHS Digital (2018) *Statistics on drug misuse England, 2018 (November update).* Available at: https://files.digital.nhs.uk/14/527824/drug-misu-eng-2018nov-rep.pdf.

Öberg, M., Jaakkola, M.S., Woodward, A., Peruga, A. & Prüss-Ustün, A. (2011) 'Worldwide burden of disease from exposure to second-hand smoke: a retrospective analysis of data from 192 countries.' *The Lancet*, 377(9760), 139–146. doi: 10.1016/S0140-6736(10)61388-8.

Office for National Statistics (2018) *Statistics on Smoking – England, 2018 [PAS].* Available at: https://digital.nhs.uk/data-and-information/publications/statistical/statistics-on-smoking/statistics-on-smoking-england-2018.

Office for National Statistics (2019) *Families and Households in the UK: 2019.* Available at: www.ons.gov.uk/peoplepopulationandcommunity/birthsdeathsandmarriages/families/bulletins/familiesandhouseholds/2019.

Ofsted (2013) *Not Yet Good Enough: Personal, Social, Health and Economic Education in Schools*, No. 130065. London: Ofsted. Available at: https://assets.publishing.service.gov.uk/government/uploads/system/uploads/attachment_data/file/413178/Not_yet_good_enough_personal__social__health_and_economic_education_in_schools.pdf.

Plan UK (2017) *Almost Half of Girls Aged 14–21 Are Embarrassed by their Periods.* Available at: https://plan-uk.org/media-centre/almost-half-of-girls-aged-14-21-are-embarrassed-by-their-periods.

Plan UK (2018) *Break the Barriers: Girls' Experiences of Menstruation in the UK.* Available at: https://plan-uk.org/file/plan-uk-break-the-barriers-report-032018pdf/download?token=Fs-HYP3v.

Public Health England (2018) *Young People's Statistics from the National Drug Treatment Monitoring System (NDTMS) 1 April 2017 to 31 March 2018.* Available at: https://assets.publishing.service.gov.uk/government/uploads/system/uploads/attachment_data/file/762446/YPStatisticsFrom-NDTMS2017to2018.pdf.

Rape and Sexual Offences (2021) *Chapter 7: Key Legislation and Offences 21 May 2021 | Legal Guidance, Sexual Offences.* Available at: www.cps.gov.uk/legal-guidance/rape-and-sexual-offences-chapter-7-key-legislation-and-offences.

Sexual Offences Act (2003, 2021) Available at: www.legislation.gov.uk/ukpga/2003/42/section/74.

The United Nations (1989) *Convention on the Rights of the Child.* Treaty Series 1577. Available at: www.unicef.org.uk/what-we-do/un-convention-child-rights.

Women's Aid (2015) *Women's Aid and Avon Launch the 'Love Don't Feel Bad' Campaign.* Available at: www.womensaid.org.uk/womens-aid-and-avon-launch-the-love-dont-feel-bad-campaign.

Women's Aid (2018) *Women's Aid Launches #LoveRespect Website for Teenage Girls at Risk of Relationship Abuse.* Available at: www.womensaid.org.uk/womens-aid-launches-loverespect-website-for-teenage-girls-at-risk-of-relationship-abuse.

Useful Resources

4Boys/4Girls Snapper Leaflet

These pocket-sized, folding paper snapper games are effective ways to reinforce learning from the *4Boys, 4Girls* booklet.

www.fpa.org.uk

Breast Self-Examination (BSE) and Testicular Self-Examination (TSE) Model

The resource contains a teen BSE and TSE model to teach young people the importance of the early detection of cancer.

www.anatomystuff.co.uk

Child Exploitation and Online Protection (CEOP)

A website for professionals and young people to report concerns and worries about online sexual abuse or the way someone has been communicating with young people online. You can make a report to one of CEOP's child protection advisors.

www.ceop.police.uk/Safety-Centre

Childline

A free, private and confidential service where young people can talk about anything. The service is available both online and on the phone, anytime.

www.childline.org.uk

Contraceptive Display Kit

The Contraceptive Display Kit is an ideal resource to facilitate thinking and talking about different methods of contraception.

www.fpa.org.uk

Coppafeel!

A breast cancer awareness charity that provides free lesson plans, resources and workshops for schools.

https://coppafeel.org

DrugWise

A useful website for reports and up-to-date information about drugs.

www.drugwise.org.uk

Equal Game Campaign

#EqualGame is UEFA's campaign to promote its vision that everyone should be able to enjoy football.

www.equalgame.com

Fink Cards

A range of conversation cards that get people talking, enhance relationships and help kids become confident communicators.

www.finkcards.com

Genderbread Person

A teaching tool for breaking the big concept of gender down into bite-sized, digestible pieces.

www.genderbread.org

Kick it Out Campaign

English football's equality and inclusion organization.

www.kickitout.org

L.E. Bowman Poetry

Author of *The Evolution of a Girl*, a collection of poetry and prose taking the reader from girl to woman; from heartbreak and anger to transformation and rebirth.

www.lebowmanpoetry.com

NHS Website

Provides free information and advice on health conditions, symptoms, healthy living, medicines and how to get help.

www.nhs.uk

R.M. Drake
A *New York Times* bestselling author; his Instagram account provides quotes for relationship education stimuli.

www.instagram.com/rmdrk

Talk to Frank
A resource for drug and alcohol topics. Find out everything you need to know about drugs, their effects and the law.

www.talktofrank.com

Teen Vogue
The young person's guide to conquering (and saving) the world. This online magazine covers the latest in celebrity news, politics, fashion, beauty, wellness and lifestyle.

www.teenvogue.com

Thinkuknow
The education programme from NCA-CEOP, a UK organization which protects children both online and offline.

www.thinkuknow.co.uk

The Equality Wheel (The Duluth Model)
This tool describes the qualities involved in healthy relationships

www.theduluthmodel.org

***The Places I've Cried in Public*, by Holly Bourne**
Young adult fiction novel tackling toxic relationships.

https://hollybourne.co.uk

Urban Dictionary
The online dictionary with definitions written by everyone. This is a great space to keep up to date with the latest slang terms relating to sex and relationships.

www.urbandictionary.com

Index